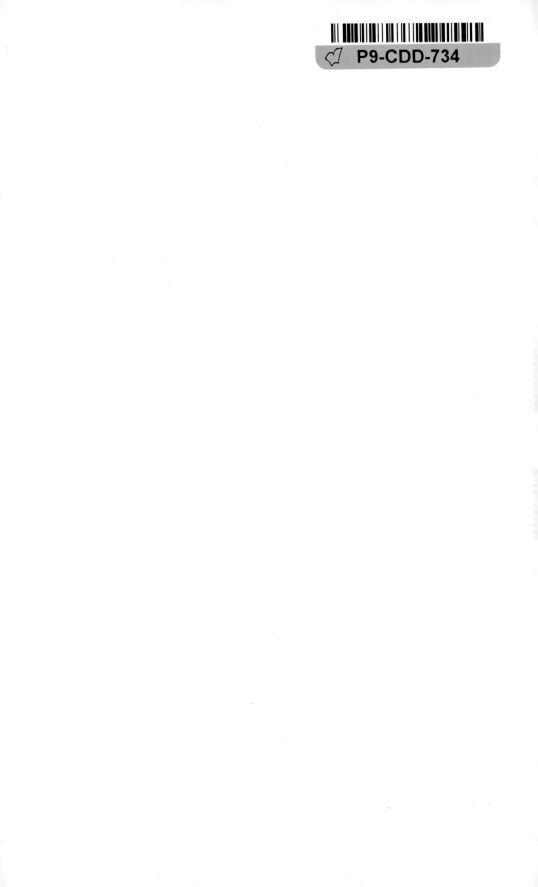

OSLER

Inspirations from a Great Physician

OSLER

Inspirations from a
Great Physician

Charles S. Bryan, M.D.

Heyward Gibbes Distinguished Professor of
Internal Medicine and Chair,
Department of Medicine,
The University of South Carolina School of Medicine,
Columbia, South Carolina

New York   Oxford
OXFORD UNIVERSITY PRESS
1997

Oxford University Press

Oxford   New York
Athens   Auckland   Bangkok   Bogota   Bombay   Buenos Aires
Calcutta   Cape Town   Dar es Salaam   Delhi   Florence   Hong Kong
Istanbul   Karachi   Kuala Lumpur   Madras   Madrid   Melbourne
Mexico City   Nairobi   Paris   Singapore   Taipei   Tokyo   Toronto

and associated companies in
Berlin   Ibadan

Library of Congress Cataloging-in-Publication Data

Bryan, Charles S.
Osler : inspirations from a great physician /
Charles S. Bryan.
p.   cm.
Includes bibliographical references and index.
ISBN 0-19-511251-2
1. Olser, William, Sir, 1849–1919—Philosophy,
2. Osler, William, Sir, 1849–1919—Influence.
I. Title.
[DNLM: 1. Osler, William, Sir, 1849–1919.
2. Physicians—biography.
WZ 100 082Ba 1997]   R464.O8B78   1997   610'.1—dc20   [B]
DNLM/DLC   for Library of Congress   96-30172

1 3 5 7 9 8 6 4 2
Printed in the United States of America
on acid-free paper

To the Memory of
Leon S. Bryan, M.D.
(1909–1972)

Preface

Men are immortalized on this earth when their good actions and qualities are imitated by those who come after. So it has been with Dr. Osler. So let it be with us.
—Philip A. Tumulty, M.D., *The Effective Clinician* (1973)

Sir William Osler (1849–1919) is the most famous and influential physician of the early twentieth century. His life can be seen in brief as the fulfillment of two dreams. As a young man he determined to become a great teacher of clinical medicine. His 1892 textbook, *The Principles and Practice of Medicine*, set a new standard and greatly advanced scientific medicine. Having realized his first dream by his early forties, he then set out, perhaps subconsciously at first, to reconcile the emerging new medical science with the old humanities. His unique blend of clinical competence, easy familiarity with the liberal arts, energy, charisma, and idealism made him something of a symbol of humanism in medicine for physicians and laypersons alike. Yet despite his fame and influence, most of today's young people, including medical students, can barely identify Osler. My purpose is to make his ideals and examples easily accessible to the present generation.

This book is based on the conviction that Osler (pronounced OH-sler) was, above all else, a motivator. He set high personal

goals, achieved them, and inspired others to do the same. Each of
the eight chapters contains a central theme: (1) time management,
(2) career planning, (3) mentoring, (4) positive thinking, (5) education, (6) caring, (7) communicating, and (8) seeking a balanced
life. Reference is made throughout the text to Osler's "Bed-Side
Library for Medical Students," which consists of ten works or
authors: the Old and New Testaments, Shakespeare, Montaigne,
Plutarch's *Lives*, Marcus Aurelius, Epictetus, Sir Thomas Browne's
Religio Medici, Cervantes's *Don Quixote*, Emerson, and Oliver
Wendell Holmes.[1] Discerning readers will find snippets here and
there based on the work of such late twentieth-century motivators
as Earl Nightingale, Brian Tracy, Dennis Waitley, Suzette Haden
Elgin, Marilyn Moats Kennedy, Wayne Dyer, and others, reflecting
a serious attempt to compare Osler's messages with theirs.[2] Researching this book, I was amazed at the extent to which Osler and
his recommended authors still deliver a relevant message. If I were
allowed to echo but one piece of Oslerian advice, my choice would
be this: "Start at once a bed-side library and spend the last half
hour of the day in communion with the saints of humanity." [3]

This book is not an attempt to fill the perceived need for a new
biography of Osler. He was almost certainly a more complicated
man than comes across in the two prize-winning volumes by
Harvey Cushing, an admiring protégé and friend chosen for the
task by Osler's widow. However, those who are largely unfamiliar
with the Osler story may find a brief outline helpful. He was born
at Bond Head Parsonage in Tecumseth Township, Upper Canada,
the eighth child and youngest son of an Anglican priest. He gradu-
ated from McGill Medical School in 1872, studied in Europe, and
returned to McGill in 1874 as an instructor in medicine. Over the
next ten years he rose rapidly in the academic ranks and in the
esteem of his colleagues while performing more than a thousand
autopsies, honing his ability to teach, and promoting goodwill and
harmony in the local medical community. In 1884 he accepted the
Chair of Clinical Medicine at the University of Pennsylvania. Five
years later he moved from Philadelphia to Baltimore to become
Chair of Medicine at the new medical school at Johns Hopkins,
and it was there that he achieved worldwide renown. Demand for
his services rose to the extent that by 1903 he suffered from what
we now call burnout. In 1905 he moved to Oxford, England, as
Regius Professor of Medicine—a prestigious job with relatively

light duties that enabled him to consolidate his reputation not only as a great clinician but also as a great humanist. In 1911 he was made a baronet and designed a coat of arms that included his famous motto, "Aequanimitas" (equanimity; calmness). The death of his son, Revere, in World War I broke his spirit, and in 1919 he died of complications of pneumonia.

So much has been written about Osler that another addition to the Osler industry requires brief justification.[4] Mine is twofold. First, each generation must understand and reinterpret charismatic figures such as Osler on its own terms. Many people today are not only unfamiliar with the context of Osler's addresses but are also uncomfortable with his highly textured prose style laced with Latin phrases and literary allusions. By placing Osler's words and deeds in a new format, I hope to encourage others to delve into the rich trove of Osleriana. Second, I believe that events and trends of the late twentieth century make Osler's message as meaningful as ever and perhaps even more so. On the centenary of Osler's birth in 1949, one of his admirers wrote: "Whatever the future holds for those engaged in the practice of medicine, the Osler message is still vital, as it carries that sweet, optimistic, courageous note which makes one glory in the day's work." [5] The extent to which this book is successful depends on whether or not I have captured that message.

Columbia, S.C.   C.S.B.

Acknowledgments

The journey that became this book began in 1962 when my father gave me his copy of *Aequanimitas*, William Osler's volume of inspirational essays. Thirty years later another aspiring undergraduate student, Ashby M. Jordan, II, inquired about a summer job and I proposed that he help me organize my thoughts about the Osler message. Silent partners during the subsequent writing of this book were members of the American Osler Society and third-year medical students at the University of South Carolina. If these students' idealism is at all representative, medicine is in good hands. This book is for them and for their generation.

I thank the following librarians: Rebecca S. Feind and George D. Terry and the staff of the Thomas Cooper Library, University of South Carolina; June Schachter and the staff of the Osler Library of the History of Medicine, McGill University, Montreal; Scott G. Marsh of the Alan Mason Chesney Archives of the History of Medicine, Johns Hopkins Medical Institutions; Kay Harwood and the staff of the Josey Health Sciences Library, Richland Memorial Hospital, Columbia, S.C.; Charles B. Greifenstein of the College of Physicians of Philadelphia; Stephen Greenberg of the National

Library of Medicine, Bethesda; and Robin Chandler of the Archives and Special Collections, Library and Center for Knowledge Management, University of California, San Francisco. Jean W. Ross carefully reviewed two versions of the manuscript and made many valuable recommendations. I thank Phillip W. Green and Bosko Postic who, as W. S. Thayer and H. A. Lafleur did for Osler during the writing of his textbook, gave able clinical help that allowed me to undertake such an ambitious project.

While assuming all responsibility for errors and shortcomings, I freely acknowledge enormous debt to the world-class Oslerians who read the entire manuscript, made many suggestions, and spared me several embarrassments. These included Richard L. Golden and Charles G. Roland as primary reviewers, Jeremiah A. Barondess, Michael Bliss, W. Bruce Fye, and Earl F. Nation. The manuscript was also critiqued by colleagues in South Carolina, including Allan S. Brett, John M. Bryan, Samuel G. Candler, Joy Drennen, Larry R. Faulkner, Frederick L. Greene, J. O'Neal Humphries, Richard A. Hoppmann, Kay F. McFarland, Elizabeth Y. Newsom, James Raymond, M. Shawn Stinson, and Harold N. Wheeler. Keith W. Davis reviewed psychological aspects, and Donald E. Saunders, Jr., allowed me to use what he calls the "scientific serenity prayer" (Chapter 6, Figure 6.1). Ward W. Briggs, Jr., and James N. Hardin translated French, German, and Latin phrases; Antonya Godbold and John Shelton provided reference assistance; and Mimi Ackerman proofread the final draft.

I am extremely grateful to Jeffrey W. House at Oxford University Press for his willingness to undertake a different kind of book. I also thank the Osler Library of the History of Medicine, McGill University, Montreal for permission to use an excerpt from one of Osler's unpublished addresses (Chapter 7); HarperCollins for permission to adapt an illustration (Figure 1.1); the Covey Leadership Center for permission to use the Time Management Matrix® (Figure 1.2); and the Osler Library at McGill, the Alan Mason Chesney Archives at Johns Hopkins, and the archives and special collections (Esther Rosencrantz Collection) at the University of California, San Francisco for permission to reproduce photographs in their collections. Finally, I thank my wife, Donna, for her support and encouragement, and my daughters, Chandlee and Emily, for their exhortation, "Keep it simple, Dad!" Whether this last advice was taken only the reader can judge.

Contents

1. Manage Time Well: *Day-Tight Compartments*   3
   Have Unifying Principles, **4** Have Definite Goals, **8**
   Plan the Day, **13** Be Methodical, **17**
   Take the Long View, **21** Study Time Management, **26**

2. Find a Calling: *Being True to Certain Ideals*   31
   Explore the Possibilities, **33** Be an Idealist, **37**
   See the Big Picture, **41** Know the History, **44**
   Join the Organizations, **48** Leave a Legacy, **53**

3. Find Mentors: *The Young Person's Friend*   59
   Begin the Journey, **60** Cultivate Teachers, **63**
   Have Heroes, **67** Take on Pupils, **72**
   Show Gratitude, **76** Understand the Chemistry, **78**

4. Be Positive: *"Prince of Friends and Benefactors"*   83

Be an Optimist, **84**   Be Generous, **88**

Work, **90**   Be Decisive, **94**

Be Tolerant of Others, **97**   Use the Mature Defenses, **100**

5. Learn and Teach: *Driving Plato's Horses*   105

Value Education, **106**   Observe and Think, **109**

Combine Principles and Practice, **115**

Be Intellectually Honest, **118**

Be Both Teacher and Student, **123**

Refine the Methods, **127**

6. Care Carefully: *The Least Sentimental and the Most Helpful*   133

Show Compassion,   **134**   Maintain Equanimity, **140**

Touch Frequently, **144**   Care for Yourself, **147**

Keep a Sense of Humor, **151**

Care for the Right Reasons, **156**

7. Communicate: *Secrets of the Heart*   161

Learn to Write, **161**   Learn to Listen, **167**

Learn to Speak, **171**   Share Concerns, **174**

Be Political, **178**   Be Careful What You Say, **182**

8. Seek Balance: *A Simple and Temperate Life*   187

Be a Good Animal, **188**   Have Family, **193**

Have Friends, **198**   Maintain Outside Interests, **202**

Answer the "Big Questions" **205**   Be Courageous **212**

Epilogue. Osler on Character: *Pursue Virtue Virtuously*   217

Notes, **221**

Index, **257**

OSLER

Inspirations from a Great Physician

1

MANAGE

TIME

WELL

Day-Tight Compartments

Is William Osler a useful role model? Our first
response is no. He was simply too good, too
talented, too productive for most of us to
emulate. Master clinician, prolific writer, pro-
moter of science, inspiring motivator, and
since his death in 1919, a durable icon of
professionalism, Osler seemingly had it all.
The historian Fielding H. Garrison called him
"one of nature's chosen" and added, "Good
looks, distinction, blithe, benignant manners,
a sunbright personality, radiant with kind feeling and good will toward his fellow men, an
Apollonian poise, swiftness and surety of
thought and speech, every gift of the gods was
his." [1] Striving to be like Osler would seem a
sure formula for failure, frustration, and damaged self-esteem.

3

Osler saw it differently. He held that he was not especially gifted. Some of those who knew him agreed; indeed, family friends held that the brightest of Canada's celebrated Osler brothers was not William but B. B.—Britton Bath Osler, the trial lawyer. Never claiming to be a scientist, William Osler made no breakthrough discoveries. Never claiming to be a scholar, he left no true literary classics. Osler confessed to Yale students what he considered to be the frank truth:

> A man who has filled Chairs in four universities, has written a successful book, and has been asked to lecture at Yale, is supposed popularly to have brains of a special quality. A few of my intimate friends really know the truth about me, as I know it! Mine, in good faith I say it, are of the most mediocre character. But what about those professorships, &c.? Just habit, a way of life, an outcome of the day's work, the vital importance of which I wish to impress upon you with all the force at my command.[2]

What, then, was his secret?

Osler combined love and tolerance for his fellow humans with industry and a set of skills now grouped and taught as "time management," broadly understood as a measured approach to life in which principles determine goals, goals determine priorities, and priorities determine what we do.[3] He taught a way of life based on "day-tight compartments," making the most of the present by blocking out the past and the future. This simple pragmatism has been criticized as shortsighted, "for the oarsmen of society; for followers rather than leaders; for carry-outers rather than decid-ers-orderers." [4] However, closer analysis reveals that Osler practiced what today's time management experts call self-unification or principle-centered living. By structuring his time according to his deepest values, he achieved both personal productivity and peace of mind. Like most great men, he excelled because he knew what he wanted and stuck to a set of well-thought-out principles.

HAVE UNIFYING PRINCIPLES

The high-sounding ideals that lace Osler's writings sometimes tempt us to dismiss him as a cardboard figure of doubtful relevance. In truth, he was a multifaceted, fun-loving, mischievous person with a healthy capacity to laugh at his own foibles and shortcomings. His early life gave little hint of the values contained in his better-known essays. Young Willie Osler lacked direction, and the result was often trouble. He totally disrupted the one-room schoolhouse in Dundas, Ontario, on at least two occasions, once by locking a flock of geese in the classroom and once by removing all of the desks and benches and hiding them in the attic. Expelled, he gleefully cried out to his sister as he rode home bareback on his father's horse, "Chattie, I've got the sack!" There followed the traditional remedy for problem pupils: boarding schools. At one, he gained notoriety as one of "Barrie's bad boys" by such feats as killing a farmer's pig with an accurately thrown stone. At another, he helped mastermind a plot whereby a disliked housekeeper was barricaded in her room and nearly asphyxiated with a burning mixture of molasses, mustard, and pepper. The *Toronto Globe* screamed, "School Row at Weston. Pupils Turn Outlaws. They Fumigate the Matron with Sulphur." [5] Only the housekeeper's lucky rescue and his brother Featherston's legal ability saved him from conviction as a felon.

Osler offset his penchant for mischief with principles gleaned as a young man from the writings of Sir Thomas Browne and Thomas Carlyle. He was introduced to Browne by the Reverend William Arthur Johnson, founder and warden of Trinity College School in Weston, Ontario. Browne was a seventeenth-century English physician who struggled with the issue of science versus faith and wrote a classic entitled *Religio Medici*. This book became Osler's guidepost to the extent that he regarded its author as his "life-long mentor." He later confided: "The Religio Medici, one of the great English classics, should be in the hands—in the hearts too—of every medical student. As I am on the confessional to-day, I may tell you that no book has had so enduring an influence on my life." [6] At age 22, he came across a pivotal passage by Thomas Carlyle, the nineteenth-century Scottish historian, philosopher, and essayist. Osler was studying for a medical school examination but having trouble concentrating because of doubts and anxieties about his future. Opening a volume of Carlyle, he read, "Our main business is not to see what lies dimly in the distance but to do what lies clearly at hand." As Osler later said, "A commonplace sentiment enough, but it hit, and stuck, and helped, and was the starting point of a habit that has enabled me to utilize to the full, the single talent entrusted to me." [7] Carlyle's sentence became Osler's credo of time management.[8] Thus Browne symbolized Osler's quest for meaning, Carlyle his quest for effectiveness, and together they formed his basis for principle-centered living in "day-tight compartments."

Principle-centered living as currently taught begins with set-ting ideals in writing. One should aim for a "major definite pur-pose," a clear statement of participation in a higher cause. Osler's major definite purpose came to be his promotion of scientific yet humanistic medicine. He stressed the value of idealism while acknowledging that as mortals we inevitably fall short: "Not that we all live up to the highest ideals, far from it—we are only men. But we have ideals, which mean much, and they are realizable, which means more." [9] At a farewell address to North American physicians on May 2, 1905, given in the ballroom of New York's Waldorf-Astoria Hotel as he prepared to leave for England and Oxford, he disclosed:

> I have had three personal ideals. One to do the day's work well and not to bother about to-morrow. It has been urged that this is not a satisfactory ideal. It is; and there is not one which the student can carry with him into practice with greater effect. To it, more than anything else, I owe whatever success I have had—to this power of settling down to the day's work and trying to do it well to the best of one's ability, and letting the future take care of itself.
>
> The second ideal has been to act the Golden Rule, as far as in me lay, towards my professional brethren and towards the patients committed to my care.
>
> And the third has been to cultivate such a measure of equanim-ity as would enable me to bear success with humility, the affection of my friends without pride and to be ready when the day of sorrow and grief came to meet it with the courage befitting a man.[10]

Osler's writings suggest that, if pressed to name his ideals, he would have added at least two more: education and persistence. Osler quoted Plato to the effect that education is essential for civilization:

> There is a shrewd remark in the *Republic* "that the most gifted minds, when they are ill-educated, become pre-eminently bad. Do not great crimes and the spirit of pure evil spring out of a fulness of

nature ruined by education rather than from any inferiority, whereas weak natures are scarcely capable of any very great good or very great evil." [11]

Here, as in many places in Osler's writings, one finds echoes of the quaint sixteenth-century prose of Sir Thomas Browne, who wrote that "we are all monsters, that is a composition of man and beast, wherein we must endeavour . . . to have the Region of Man above that of Beast, and sense to sit but at the feet of reason." [12] Osler insisted on higher standards of education for physicians:

> The higher the standard of education in a profession the less marked will be the charlatanism, whereas no greater incentive to its development can be found than in sending out from our colleges men who have not had mental training sufficient to enable them to judge between the excellent and the inferior, the sound and the unsound, the true and the half true. [13]

Moreover:

> The commonest as well as the saddest mistake is to mistake one's profession, and this we doctors do often enough, some of us, without knowing it. There are men who have never had the preliminary education which would enable them to grasp the fundamental truths of the science on which medicine is based. . . . There are only two sorts of doctors; those who practise with their brains, and those who practise with their tongues. [14]

He also valued persistence and work, which he called "the master-word in medicine." Both were necessary: "Ten years' hard work tells with colleagues and friends in the profession, and with enlarged clinical facilities the physician enters upon the second, or bread-and-butter period." [15] In 1897 he suggested:

> A young fellow with staying powers who avoids entanglements, may look forward in twenty years to a good consultation practice in any town of 40,000 to 50,000 inhabitants. Some such man, perhaps, in a town far distant, taking care of his education, and not of his bank book, may be the Austin Flint [1812–1886; a leading physician and textbook author] of New York in 1930. [16]

In summary, his major unifying principles included living in day-tight compartments, following the Golden Rule, cultivating equanimity, valuing education, and working diligently toward clear-cut goals; he was people-oriented and principle-centered.

But what about personal ambition? Ralph Waldo Emerson, one of the authors in Osler's recommended bedside library, is often remembered for having written the aphorism "Hitch your wagon to a star." The context of Emerson's famous exhortation, however, was the need not for great personal ambition but rather for lofty principles:

> All our social and political action leans on principles. To accomplish anything excellent the will must work for catholic and universal ends. . . . Gibraltar may be strong, but ideas are impregnable, and bestow on the hero their invincibility. . . . Hitch your wagon to a star. Let us not fag in paltry works which serve our pot and bag alone. . . . Work rather for those interests which the divinities honor and promote,—justice, love, freedom, knowledge, utility.[17]

As to where to look for principles, Osler's conventional answer was Scripture and the great minds of the ages. He strongly recommended honing principles through regular bedtime reading from the works of those "saints of humanity" who have left us the classics of literature. He told students:

> The all-important thing is to get a relish for the good company of the race in a daily intercourse with some of the great minds of all ages. Now, in the spring-time of life, pick your intimates among them, and begin a systematic cultivation of their works. . . . Start at once a bed-side library and spend the last half hour of the day in communion with the saints of humanity.[18]

Reflection on basic principles promotes "the calm life" necessary for sustained pursuit of high goals: "The truth that lowliness is young ambition's ladder is hard to grasp, and when accepted harder to maintain. It is so difficult to be still amidst bustle, to be quiet amidst noise; yet . . . the calm life [is] necessary to continuous work for a high purpose."[19] Osler realized that the inner calm that precedes outward equanimity results from a way of life rooted in definite principles, clear goals, a daily action plan, and determination.

HAVE DEFINITE GOALS

Like most high achievers, Osler was an obsessive goal-setter who viewed life predominantly as an unbroken series of projects. Today's time-management experts advise that we should set in writing long-range, intermediate, and short-term goals that are consistent with our unifying principles (Figure 1.1). Numerous studies suggest that those people who keep written goals (fewer than five percent of the population) obtain a disproportionately large share of the good things that life has to offer, however measured. Most experts recommend keeping long-term goals largely to ourselves, and whether Osler maintained written goals is not known. However, he clearly understood their importance: "The direction of our vision is everything." [20] Sir Thomas Browne had said, "In this virtuous Voyage of thy Life hull not about like the Ark without the use of Rudder, Mast, or Sail, and bound for no Port." [21] Written goals provide the reassurance and resolve to proceed with confidence and optimism even when the winds seem unfavorable. And as Osler put it, "When schemes are laid in advance, it is surprising how often the circumstances fit in with them." [22]

What were Osler's career goals? He started out to be a clergyman but concluded after one year at Trinity College that he would

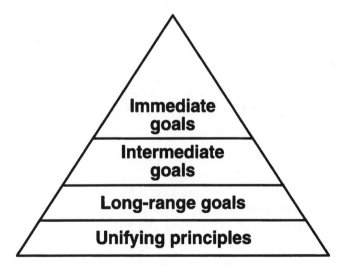

Figure 1.1. Time management as a hierarchy of goals based on principles. (Adapted from Hobbs, 1987).

rather study medicine. After receiving his medical degree, he went abroad—with financial help from his brother E. B. (Edmund Boyd Osler, the financier)—to study physiology and pathology in London, Paris, Vienna, and Berlin. But what would be his eventual field? He strongly considered ophthalmology. Then he received a letter from Dr. R. Palmer Howard, a mentor, informing him that other candidates and specifically one Frank Buller were better qualified for the ophthalmology training position in Montreal. Howard advised Osler to try instead to "cultivate the whole field" of medicine in order to become an outstanding generalist physician. This was discouraging advice:

> As you may imagine I was not a little disappointed at the blighting of my prospects as an ophthalmic surgeon, but I accept the inevitable with a good grace. . . . I had hoped in an ophthalmic practice to have a considerable amount of time at my disposal, and a fair return in a shorter time, but in a general practice which will be much slower to obtain (if it becomes of any size) what ever time you may have is always liable to be broken in upon.[23]

In Berlin he met the great pathologist Rudolph Virchow, and it was then and there that he resolved to become a great clinician and teacher.[24] Years later, as he was about to leave North America for England, Osler confided that his aim all along had been

> to be ranked with the men who have done so much for the profession in this country—to rank in the class of Nathan Smith, Bartlett, James Jackson, Bigelow, Alonzo Clark, Metcalf, W. W. Gerhard, Draper, Pepper, DaCosta, and others. The chief desire of my life has been to become a clinician of the same stamp with these great men, whose names we all revere and who did so much good work for clinical medicine.[25]

In 1874 Osler returned to McGill with this goal in mind.

To be proficient at all of medicine was a daunting task, even back then. Osler made the autopsy room his main laboratory. He spent countless hours carrying out meticulous dissections, recording his findings, and correlating the results with the patients' clinical records. As the days became months and the months became years, his proficiency increased and he acquired a large local reputation. Then came the opportunity to become Chair of Clinical Medicine at the University of Pennsylvania, a prestigious position that would enhance his reputation and sphere of influence. Should he leave his native Canada? Osler knew that he had to go if he were to achieve his goal of ranking among the giants of the medical world. When he left McGill, the students went down to the railway station to see him off. One of them recalled that Osler "walked up and down the platform, trying to express his regret at leaving us, but finished by saying—'Gentlemen—there is no use talking. I must admit that I am leaving McGill for a larger field through *ambition*.' " [26]

Written goals reinforce the resolve or "tenacity of will" to leave our comfort zones for a higher cause:

> To few is given the tenacity of will which enables a man to pursue a cherished purpose through a quarter of a century . . . to fewer still is the fruition granted. Too often the reaper is not the sower. Too often the fate of those who labour at some object for the public good is to see their work pass into other hands.[27]

But since our highest goals should be founded in causes that transcend our own well-being, we should rejoice when our efforts "pass into other hands." Goals that are largely self-serving can bring short-term success but all too frequently culminate in bitter disappointment. Clear goals not only inspire but also liberate, because they allow us to say no to others' requests that, while legitimate, don't match our own priorities. This principle explains the observation by a physician in rural Maryland that he could not get Osler to come from Baltimore to see a patient even for a large consultation fee but could always get him to come for an interesting autopsy.[28] A consultation might help one sick person and earn him money, but would do little to further his becoming a master teacher. However, an interesting autopsy would increase his fund of solid information and was therefore more consistent with his long-term goals.

Osler also understood that we must set goals carefully because we are likely to reach them. He warned young physicians that financial success should not be their primary concern:

> In a play of Oscar Wilde's one of the characters remarks, "there are only two great tragedies in life, not getting what you want—and getting it!" and I have known consultants whose treadmill life illustrated the bitterness of this *mot*, and whose great success at sixty did not bring the comfort they had anticipated at forty. The

mournful echo of the words of the preacher rings in their ears, words which I not long ago heard quoted with deep feeling by a distinguished physician, "Better is an handful with quietness, than both the hands full with travail and vexation of spirit." [29]

Moreover:

Now, while nothing disturbs our mental placidity more sadly than straightened means, and the lack of those things after which the Gentiles seek, I would warn you against the trials of the day soon to come to some of you—the day of large and successful practice. Engrossed late and soon in professional cares, getting and spending, you may so lay waste your powers that you may find, too late, with hearts given away, that there is no place in your habit-stricken souls for those gentler influences which make life worth living.[30]

Osler "had the greatest contempt for the doctor who made financial gain the first object of his work" and "even seemed to go so far as to think that a man could not make more than a bare living and still be an honest and competent physician." [31] Our best protections against what Osler called "the corroding influence of mammon" are high standards and high purpose, for

in the enormous development of material interests there is danger lest we miss altogether the secret of a nation's life, the true test of which is to be found in its intellectual and moral standards. There is no more potent antidote to the corroding influence of mammon than the presence in a community of a body of men devoted to science, living for investigation and caring nothing for the lust of the eyes and the pride of life.[32]

Although financial self-interest must be tempered by values, Osler underscored that it is not our principles and goals but rather our actions that define us:

Thucydides [the Greek historian] it was who said of the Greeks that they possessed "the power of thinking before they acted, and of acting too." The same is true in a high degree of the English race. To know just what has to be done, then do it, comprises the whole philosophy of practical life.[33]

Osler's life illustrates the truism that we must dream to decide what we want, and then work toward long-term goals through daily actions based on principles.

PLAN THE DAY

Osler's preferred daily routine contained at least three elements: interacting with people, working on one or more projects, and contemplating the meaning of life through communion with "the saints of humanity." He insisted, "When the day's activities are properly divided and rightly balanced, work is not work, but pleasure." [34] Whether he wrote out a plan for each day the night before, as is now recommended, is not known. However, his philosophy of "day-tight compartments" accords with the advice given by today's time-management experts.

The famous metaphor came from the watertight compartments that protected the great ocean liners of Osler's era:

> I stood on the bridge of one of the great liners, ploughing the ocean at 25 knots. "She is alive," said my companion, "in every plate; a huge monster with brain and nerves, an immense stomach, a wonderful heart and lungs, and a splendid system of locomotion." Just at that moment a signal sounded, and all over the ship the watertight compartments were closed. "Our chief factor of safety," said the Captain. "In spite of the *Titanic*," I said. "Yes," he replied, "in spite of the *Titanic*." Now each of you is a much more marvellous organization than the great liner, and bound on a longer voyage. What I urge is that you so learn to control the machinery as to live with "day-tight compartments" as the most certain way to ensure safety on the voyage. Get on the bridge, and see that at least the great bulkheads are in working order. Touch a button and hear, at every level of your life, the iron doors shutting out the Past—the dead yesterdays. Touch another and shut off, with a metal curtain, the Future—the unborn to-morrows. Then you are safe—safe for to-day![35]

Osler emphasized, "Shut off the past! Let the dead past bury its dead. So easy to say, so hard to realize! The truth is, the past haunts us like a shadow. To disregard it is not easy." [36] It is even more difficult to block out the future:

> The load of to-morrow, added to that of yesterday, carried to-day makes the strongest falter. Shut off the future as tightly as the past. No dreams, no visions, no delicious fantasies, no castles in the air, with which, as the old song so truly says, "hearts are broken, heads are turned." To youth, we are told, belongs the future, but the wretched to-morrow that so plagues some of us has no cer-

tainty, except through to-day. Who can tell what a day may bring forth? . . . The future is to-day—there is no to-morrow! The day of a man's salvation is *now*—the life of the present, of to-day, lived earnestly, intently, without a forward-looking thought, is the only insurance for the future. Let the limit of your horizon be a twenty-four-hour circle.[37]

He urged medical students:

Throw away . . . all ambition beyond that of doing the day's work well. The travellers on the road to success live in the present, heedless of taking thought for the morrow, having been able at some time, and in some form or other, to receive into their heart of hearts this maxim of the Sage of Chelsea [Thomas Carlyle]: Your business is "not to *see* what lies dimly at a distance, but to *do* what lies clearly at hand." [38]

He added:

The quiet life in day-tight compartments will help you to bear your own and others' burdens with a light heart. Pay no heed to the Batrachians [frogs and toads] who sit croaking idly by the stream. Life is a straight, plain business, and the way is clear, blazed for you by generations of strong men, into whose labours you enter and whose ideals must be your inspiration.[39]

But it was crucial to bring a routine to this concept of daily living:

I appeal to the freshmen especially, because you to-day make a beginning, and your future career depends very much upon the habits you will form during this session. To follow the routine of the classes is easy enough, but to take routine into every part of your daily life is a hard task.

Osler apparently recognized intuitively that life in day-tight compartments presupposes goals, planning, and effective routines.

Osler's emphasis on habits and routines made allowance for the anxiety and depression that are part and parcel of the adventuresome life. Drawing from John Bunyan's *Pilgrim's Progress*, an allegorical story of a man's journey to the Promised Land, he suggested:

Some of you will start out joyfully as did Christian and Hopeful, and for many days will journey safely towards the Delectable Mountains, dreaming of them and not thinking of disaster until you find yourselves in the strong captivity of Doubt and under the grinding tyranny of Despair. . . . No student escapes wholly from these perils and trials; be not disheartened; expect them.

But the best protection against doubt and despair, or anxiety and depression, is good time management:

Let each hour of the day have its allotted duty, and cultivate that power of concentration which grows with its exercise, so that the attention neither flags nor wavers, but settles with a bull-dog tenacity on the subject before you. Constant repetition makes a good habit fit easily in your mind, and by the end of the session you may have gained that most precious of all knowledge—the power to work.[40]

His advice was to plan the day, then live in the present:

As to your method of work, I have a single bit of advice, which I give with the earnest conviction of its paramount influence in any success which may have attended my efforts in life—*Take no thought for the morrow.* Live neither in the past nor in the future, but let each day's work absorb your entire energies, and satisfy your widest ambition. . . . The student who is worrying about his future, anxious over the examinations, doubting his fitness for the profession, is certain not to do so well as the man who cares for nothing but the matter in hand, and who knows not whither he is going![41]

Harvey Cushing, Osler's biographer, observed that it "was not in Osler's make-up to worry." [42] Osler knew that worry—as opposed to planning—is counterproductive.

Osler's daily routine during a 1905 ocean voyage to England illustrates his ability to structure his time through planning. He had reading to do and projects to finish, but he also wanted to relate to the other passengers and especially to the physicians on board. His solution was to organize his books and papers, rise early, read for four to five hours, and then work on a paper that he was writing. At noon, he surfaced on the deck "free from care, the liveliest person aboard." He merrily led the small group of physicians on board to form a "North Atlantic Medical Society" that met every afternoon for tea, fellowship, and fictitious case reports designed to elicit hearty laughs.[43] Thus he struck a happy balance between solitude and sociability. By structuring his time carefully, he had enough for his own projects and enough to share with others. Planning made it look easy.

At no time was Osler's ability to plan the day more evident than while he was writing his textbook, *The Principles and Practice of Medicine*. It was the textbook that would spread his reputation far beyond the places where he had taught—Montreal, Philadelphia, and Baltimore—and thus help him consummate his ambition to be recognized as a great clinician-teacher. He had done the necessary groundwork. But how could he find time to write the massive book, especially without a sabbatical? The year was 1891. Osler was in Baltimore as Chair of Medicine at Johns Hopkins. Financial constraints had delayed the school's opening, so he was not yet responsible for medical students. Capable subordinates could handle the clinical responsibilities. Osler had a window of opportunity and understood that it was now or never. He obtained a contract with a publisher. But like most writers, he found the initial going slow. And so he set new priorities and established a routine:

> Early in May I gave up the house, 209 Monument St., and went to my rooms at the Hospital. The routine there was:—8 a.m. to 1 p.m. dictation, 2 p.m. visit to the private patients and special cases in the wards, after which revision, &c. After 5 p.m. I saw my outside cases; dined at the club about 6:30, loafed until 9:30, bed at 10, up at 7 a.m. . . . During the writing of the work I lost only one afternoon through transient indisposition and never a night's rest. Between September 1890 and January 1892 I gained nearly eight lbs. in weight.[44]

This terse account offers several insights. By giving up his home, he eliminated the hassles of housekeeping and the need to travel back and forth. He structured his time in such a way that his days quickly assumed a rhythm. He avoided the guilt trap of having to work constantly, recognizing that for peak performance one should balance periods of total focus with down time or time out.[45] And he slept well because, having organized his time, he freed himself from the diffuse anxiety that goes with feeling pressured. Planning the day in advance is useful prophylaxis against insomnia—much of which is due to worrying about whether we'll forget something the next day. Osler thus intuitively grasped the essence of a time-management system based on principles, goals, and action steps. His principle might have been "to promote medical education," his long-term goal "to be a clinician-teacher of the first rank," his intermediate goal "to complete a textbook of medicine by early 1892," and a representative daily goal "to complete the third revision of the first section of chapter five." Soon his colleague William H. Welch exulted, "Osler is in labor; a book is born."

Osler's ability to focus was impressive. The hospital superintendent, Henry Hurd, later marveled:

> I have never known any man who had such an ability to do steady, regular and grinding work day after day and week after week as he displayed during the period he was writing his text-book on medicine. He arose early in the morning and remained at his work at every leisure moment not required by medical duties. He filled his room with all sorts of medical literature and consulted every necessary work . . . and after a labour of seven months, he finished his gigantic task, which will always be a monument to his ability as a writer and to his knowledge as a physician.[46]

The textbook was an immediate success, and its influence extended even beyond medical circles. In 1897, a Baptist minister named Frederick T. Gates took the book with him on a summer vacation to the Catskill Mountains and was enthralled not only by the charm and power of Osler's writing but also by the potentials of scientific medicine. Gates was an adviser to John D. Rockefeller, whom he persuaded to invest in medical education and research. The result had far-reaching impact both on medical education in the United States and on international health.[47]

BE METHODICAL

Contemporaries marveled at Osler's ability to work rapidly and effectively. Again and again, other physicians asked, "How does he do it?"[48] Osler's answer was simple: method and thoroughness. A colleague from his school days confirmed that "Osler never did anything by halves" and that he "was more regular and systematic than words can say; in fact, it was hardly necessary, living in the house with him, to have a time-piece of one's own. One could tell the time exactly from his movements from the hour of his rising at seven-thirty until he turned out his light at eleven o'clock."[49] Others made the same observation; for instance, a student at Oxford observed that "you had to make an early start for at the tick of nine

Dr. Osler was at the door of the ward and all work stopped." [50] He
seemed to have a built-in clock and he did not waste time.

Osler hurried but did not show the hurry sickness exemplified
by what we have come to know as the type A personality. In
Montreal it was noted that he "always seemed to be in a hurry to
get somewhere. As a boy I remember admiring his personal appearance with his high silk hat and his Prince Albert coat. He knew all
the children on the street and had a cheery word for them." [51] In
Baltimore it was remembered that each morning, "a few minutes
before nine he entered the hospital door" and "humming gaily,
with arm passed through that of his assistant, he started with brisk,
springing step down the corridor towards the wards." [52] These
observations confirm that Osler somehow worked fast yet remained sensitive to those around him. Marian Osborne, his niece,
once remarked that she said, "Hurry, Hurry, we shall be late." Osler
replied: "Hurry? Never hurry—hurry is the devil. More people [are]
killed by hurry than by disease." [53]

Osler valued method more than speed and taught that without
method only the most brilliant can succeed: "Ask of any active business man or a leader in a profession the secret which enables him to
accomplish much work, and he will reply in one word, *system*; or as I
shall term it, the *Virtue of Method*, the harness without which only
the horses of genius travel." [54] He may have learned the increasing
importance of good habits as one grows older from his shadow presence, Sir Thomas Browne: "But age does not rectify, but incurvates
our natures, turning bad dispositions into worse habits, and (like
diseases) brings on incurable vices; for every day as we grow weaker
in age, we grow stronger in sin, and the number of our days does but
make our sins innumerable." [55] Yet he held that method was but one
of four qualities requisite for success in medicine:

> The Art of Detachment, the Virtue of Method, and the Quality of
> Thoroughness may make you students, in the true sense of the
> word, successful practitioners, or even great investigators; but your
> characters may still lack that which can alone give permanence to
> powers—the *Grace of Humility*.[56]

Detachment is useful for goal-setting while method and thoroughness promote goal-accomplishment, which builds self-esteem. Humility helps us work with others, multiplying our effectiveness.
Charles R. Hobbs writes, "Show me a person with high self-esteem

and humility, and you will show me an effective manager of time, a tremendously powerful individual." [57] Such a person was William Osler.

Although Osler knew and taught the benefits of being well-organized and time-efficient, he also knew that these traits do not come easily. He asked students, "How can you take the greatest possible advantage of your capacities with the least possible strain? By cultivating system. I say cultivating advisedly, since some of you will find the acquisition of systematic habits very hard." [58] Being systematic distinguishes the successful person from the dilettante:

> Thoroughness is the most difficult habit to acquire, but it is the pearl of great price, worth all the worry and trouble of the search. The dilettante lives an easy, butterfly life, knowing nothing of the toil and labour with which the treasures of knowledge are dug out of the past, or wrung by patient research in the laboratories. [59]

In 1877, when Osler was only 28, he told medical students at McGill:

> Now let me add a word of advice on the method of studying. The secret of successful working lies in the systematic arrangement of what you have to do, and in the methodical performance of it. With all of you this is possible, for few disturbing elements exist in the student's life to interrupt the allotted duty which each hour of the day should possess. Make out, each one for himself, a time-table, with the hours of lecture, study, and recreation, and follow closely and conscientiously the programme there indicated. I know of no better way to accomplish a large amount of work, and it saves the mental worry and anxiety which will surely haunt you if your tasks are done in an irregular and desultory way. With too many, unfortunately, working habits are not cultivated until the constraining dread of an examination is felt. [60]

In medicine, as in other walks of life, being systematic entails attention to detail that inevitably improves ability:

> Faithfulness in the day of small things will insensibly widen your powers, correct your faculties, and, in moments of despondency, comfort may be derived from a knowledge that some of the best work of the profession has come from men whose clinical field was limited but well-tilled. The important thing is to make the lesson of each case tell on your education. The value of experience is not in seeing much, but in seeing wisely. [61]

A systematic approach is the best way to keep up with one's reading, which in turn is essential to mastering medicine or any other subject:

> Effort and system gradually train a man's capacity to read intelligently and profitably, but only while the green years are on his head is the habit to be acquired, and in a desultory life, without fixed hours, and with his time at the beck and call of everybody, a man needs a good deal of reserve and determination to maintain it. Once the machinery is started, the effort is not felt in the keen interest in a subject. As Aristotle remarks, "In the case of our habits we are only masters of the beginning, their growth by gradual stages being imperceptible, like the growth of a disease"; and so it is with this habit of reading, of which you are only master at the beginning— once acquired, you are its slave.[62]

Osler recognized that punctuality and reliability win far more friends and respect than do charm and glibness. Indeed, he held that physicians should be punctual and should speak concisely, and that these two attributes—both reflecting self-discipline based on principles of time management—would do much to compensate for other shortcomings.[63]

Like all masters of time management, Osler taught the necessity of good habits:

> A few years ago a Xmas card went the rounds, with the legend "Life is just one 'derned' thing after another," which, in more refined language, is the same as saying "Life is a habit," a succession of actions that become more or less automatic. This great truth, which lies at the basis of all actions, muscular or psychic, is the keystone of the teaching of Aristotle, to whom the formation of habits was the basis of moral excellence. "In a word, habits of any kind are the result of actions of the same kind; and so what we have to do, is to give a certain character to these particular actions." (*Ethics* [Aristotle]). . . . The same great law reaches through mental and moral states. "Character," which partakes of both, in Plutarch's words, is "long-standing habit." [64]

He taught that time management should be an ingrained habit:

> Control of the mind as a working machine, the adaptation in it of habit, so that its action becomes almost as automatic as walking, is the end of education—and yet how rarely reached! It can be accomplished with deliberation and repose, never with hurry and worry. Re-

alize how much time there is, how long the day is. Realize that you have sixteen waking hours, three or four of which at least should be devoted to making a silent conquest of your mental machinery.[65]

He practiced what he preached in this regard. Thus Wilder Penfield, a medical student at Oxford, observed that Osler "frequently left the dinner table before coffee was served to retire to his library but he never worked late at night. He often emerged in the middle of the evening to talk for awhile, and regularly at ten o'clock, he was in bed." [66] Osler jealously guarded his time for regular reading and writing, knowing that those vital activities would be the first to be crowded out should he fail to structure his time in advance.

Osler admired others who managed time effectively. For example, he praised the physician Alfred Stillé for his "method and accuracy" and for "the lesson of a long and good life. It is contained in a sentence of his Valedictory Address: *'Only two things are essential, to live uprightly and to be wisely industrious.'* " [67] However, being wisely industrious by no means implies that we should resemble robots. Thus in praising Edward Livingston Trudeau, the founder of the tuberculosis sanatorium movement in the United States, Osler quoted from one of Trudeau's letters to the effect that in becoming efficiency experts we should never block out emotion and feeling: "Are there no other ideals than efficiency and success? I know you hate sentiment; but with some of us sentiment stands for a good deal and is a real factor in the problems of life." [68] Osler's ability to enthuse and to influence individuals, groups, and indeed an entire profession attests to his ability to be methodical yet show human concern at the same time. Harvey Cushing remarked of Osler that although the ability to secure others' cooperation "is of course the great secret of getting things done in the world, as many know . . . he practised it, as many do not." [69] Osler realized that effective time management, far from being self-centered, liberates us to work with others more effectively.

TAKE THE LONG VIEW

The young William Osler was "very much like most normal men, save in the possession of an unusual charm, and of an initiative and foresight uncommonly developed." [70] His sequential long-term goals were to master human pathology and clinical medicine, to achieve stature as a medical educator, to become a medical statesman, and to consolidate as a legacy a large personal library. Although he spent several hours each day toward the attainment of a long-term goal, he also gave priority to the people in his life. In this and in other ways, he showed that perspective comes from taking the long view.

Osler emphasized that we must step back from time to time: "A rare and precious gift is the Art of Detachment, by which a man may so separate himself from a life-long environment as to take a panoramic view of the conditions under which he has lived and moved: it frees him from Plato's den long enough to see the realities as they are, the shadows as they appear." [71] He told a graduating class of nursing students that the history of humankind often forms a dismal record:

> In the gradual division of labour, by which civilization has emerged from barbarism, the doctor and the nurse have been evolved, as useful accessories in the incessant warfare in which man is en- gaged. The history of the race is a grim record of passions and ambitions, of weaknesses and vanities, a record, too often, of bar- baric inhumanity, and even to-day, when philosophers would have us believe his thoughts had widened, he is ready as of old to shut the gates of mercy, and to let loose the dogs of war. It was in one of these attacks of race-mania that your profession, until then unset- tled and ill-defined, took, under Florence Nightingale—ever blessed be her name—its modern position. [72]

Broad-mindedness allows us to transcend these limitations: "The great minds, the great works transcend all limitations of time, of language, and of race, and the scholar can never feel initiated into the company of the elect until he can approach all of life's prob- lems from the cosmopolitan standpoint." [73] Still, Osler acknow- ledged that it is often difficult to be objective about the course of our own lives:

> From two points of view alone have we a wide and satisfactory view of life—one, as, amid the glorious tints of the early morn, ere the dew of youth has been brushed off, we stand at the foot of the hill, eager for the journey; the other, wider, perhaps less satisfactory, as we gaze from the summit, at the lengthening shadows cast by the

setting sun. From no point in the ascent have we the same broad outlook, for the steep and broken pathway affords few halting places with an unobscured view.[74]

If he understood the difficulty of achieving proper perspective, he also knew that if one does the little things well, the larger issues have a way of taking care of themselves. He noted that "William James made a remark that clung—'We live forward, we understand backwards. The philosophers tell us that there is no present, no now—the fleeting moment was as we try to catch it.'"[75] Osler was usually decisive, often making big decisions with remarkable speed, because he was clear about his principles and goals and had a good sense of what was important and what was urgent.

Stephen R. Covey, chairman and founder of the Covey Leadership Center, and his colleagues suggest that all activities fall into one of four categories based on whether they are important and whether they are urgent. Some things are both urgent and important; some are urgent but not important; some are important but not urgent; and some are neither important nor urgent (see Figure 1.2).[76] Most people, when asked in which category one should concentrate, answer that top priority should logically go to those matters that are both urgent and important (quadrant I in Figure 1.2). However, long-term success and happiness depend on successful completion of matters that are important but not urgent (quadrant II in Figure 1.2). The things that matter most—for example, health, family, friendships, finances, education, hobbies, and intellectual and spiritual growth—seldom demand top priority on a given day. Yet it is in quadrant II that we generally realize the truth of the Pareto principle (named after the Italian economist Vilfredo Pareto): 80 percent of results derive from 20 percent of activities. The extent to which we focus on quadrant II activities day in and day out determines whether we succeed or fail, and to what extent.

Examination of Osler's life reveals that he instinctively understood this principle. He knew to concentrate most of his effort on quadrant II, deal with quadrant I matters as they arose, cope with quadrant III matters as efficiently as possible, and delete quadrant IV matters from further consideration. For example, his Johns Hopkins colleague William Sydney Thayer observed of

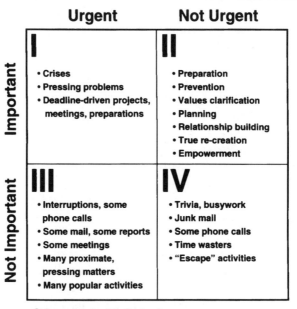

Figure 1.2. The Time Management Matrix® in which activities are categorized on the basis of importance and urgency (Reproduced with permission of Covey Leadership Center, Inc., 3507 N. University Ave., P.O. Box 19008, Provo, Utah, 84604-4479).

Osler, "For the great world he had no time. He gave none to society. But at medical meetings and at gatherings of his colleagues, he was a constant attendant and a central figure. Too often these gatherings trailed on to late hours, but before one knew it, by ten o'clock he was gone." [77] Having many social contacts was neither urgent nor important to Osler. Having a few close friends and innumerable warm acquaintances within the medical profession was not urgent on any given day but was of major long-term importance. Therefore he faithfully attended medical meetings—yet not to the extent that his time for other things would be usurped. He understood the importance of what might be called quadrant II living.

Osler's grasp of this concept can be illustrated by two episodes that occurred while he was writing *The Principles and Practice of Medicine*. Writing the textbook was a quadrant II priority. Although extremely important to his long-term goals, it was not a matter of urgency at any particular time. Yet how should he manage time-consuming interruptions in a way that did not offend the people in his life?

In the first episode, Osler was walking down a corridor of the Johns Hopkins Hospital when he encountered a former student from McGill University. The student had not seen Osler for nearly ten years and had not stood out in the class. There had even been another student in the class by the same name. Introducing himself to Osler, the young man said apologetically, "Of course you don't remember me."

"Remember you?" Osler beamed: "You're *Arthur J.* MacD—, McGill, 1882. Come with me, I've something to show you and then we'll go to lunch." [78] Hardly missing a stride, Osler took the young man by the arm and embraced him into his own schedule. Almost instantaneously, Osler gave quadrant I status to what many people might consider a quadrant III interruption, because affirming the people in his life was a top priority. But he did it in a time-efficient manner that served both parties. The young man received an enormous affirmation, and Osler was able to return to working on the textbook on schedule.

In the second example of how Osler applied this concept, his main concern one Sunday afternoon in August 1891 was to give parting advice to two young physicians, George Dock and Henri A. Lafleur, who were about to become professors at other medical schools. As the three men entered the Maryland Club for lunch, Osler was handed a telegram announcing the death of a former Montreal colleague, Dr. Richard Lea MacDonnell. It was a blow to Osler, but he proceeded to entertain his young friends as though little or nothing had happened. As they returned to their rooms at the hospital, Osler casually asked Lafleur if he might borrow his copy of John Keats's poem "In Memoriam." Later that afternoon, the three men met in the hospital lobby and headed back toward the Maryland Club. At the first street corner, Osler handed an envelope to Dock, who was closest to the mailbox. Dock observed that the letter was addressed to the editor of the *New York Medical Journal*.

A short while later, Dock found an obituary of MacDonnell in the same journal—unsigned but clearly written by Osler. Dock then realized that in little more than two hours on a hot Sunday afternoon in Baltimore, Osler had written an obituary of nearly 500 words, considered one quotation and chosen another, finished the manuscript, and mailed it. By making the obituary a quadrant I matter, he had avoided procrastination and was able to return to the textbook. And he did this without mentioning it at all to the two young men, who felt that they were the sole objects of his attention that Sunday afternoon.[79]

Such episodes were apparently typical of Osler. Cushing marveled that it was "difficult to understand how he found time to read and where he did all his writing," adding that Osler "knew how to capture the moment." Osler was seldom annoyed by interruptions; he was "ready to give freely of his time to another" and gave the appearance of being "the most care-free of mortals." [80] He recognized that one has little control over external events and other people's expectations. But despite distractions, one can move toward goals by setting clear principles and priorities. Osler, like many highly productive people, developed the ability to set short-range goals almost instantaneously. By taking the long view, he achieved not only personal productivity but also wide influence among his contemporaries.

STUDY TIME MANAGEMENT

Osler seems to have been a serious student of time management. His cousin Marian Osborne observed that she "never saw him idle or sleeping in the day-time, or sitting staring into space. The day always seemed too short for him to accomplish all he desired even with his boundless energy and his system of work." [81] Thayer observed, "He utilized every minute of his time. . . . On railway, in cab, on his way to and from consultations, in tramways, and in the old 'bob-tailed' car that used to carry us to the hospital, book and pencil were ever in his hand, and wherever he was, the happy thought was caught on the wing and noted down." [82] Cushing mused that "Osler's calendar was like india-rubber and could be thus stretched without apparent loss of time for other things." [83] Curiously, Osler was somewhat slow to adopt some of the time-saving devices that were available to him. He privately protested the installation of telephones in physicians' offices and seldom used a carriage to go from place to place. Nevertheless, it is obvious from remarks made by and about Osler that he regarded efficiency as a skill that, like any other, must be constantly honed.

Osler usually managed to keep others from monopolizing his time without offending them. One Baltimore physician noted not only that "Dr. Osler lost less time than any person we have known" but also that he "never allowed anyone to waste it for him." [84] Thayer observed that "no one could speak consecutively to Osler against his will." [85] He also paraphrased Osler's advice concerning how to avoid time-wasting conversations: "Save the fleeting minute; do not stop by the way. Learn gracefully to dodge the bore. Strike first and quickly, and before he has recovered from the blow, be gone; 'tis the only way." [86] On ward rounds, Osler focused on what mattered without getting bogged down in talk:

> In a large private ward service it was not possible for him to spend a long time with each patient. To his house officers it was always a source of interest and a good lesson to observe how he could get into and out of a patient's room without giving a chance for the flood-gates of talk to open. Many patients would lament that they had not been able to tell him this or that. But with this he had a remarkable ability in discerning when the patient needed a special interview and he was always ready to give it.[87]

He disliked long conversations and long letters. He once wrote across a multipage letter from a patient, "Please return summarized." [88]

Cushing notes that although Osler was "essentially sociable," he nevertheless "had the great gift of appearing to be longer in company than he really was; of being able to fraternize briefly and to withdraw without his withdrawal being pointed." [89] Thus he would breeze into the room where his wife was serving tea, charm everyone present, and then within 15 minutes "he was off." [90] His excuse for leaving would often be "an important engagement" that turned out to be the reading room of a medical library.[91] Osler was not hesitant to assert his right to control his time. Once, for example, a self-important professor from a distant medical school showed up unexpectedly at Osler's private clinic. The professor later recalled, "I found him delightful, but after a few minutes I was bowed out of the room in a most positive manner. Later I thought I ought to get angry about it but I couldn't; he was so nice about it all and I can see that he was right." [92] Osler later went out of his way to accommodate the visitor, but on his own terms. He knew how to suggest that it was time for people to leave without offending them.

Osler stressed the value of time management to his medical students. Many of them heard him say in his "round the table talks" in Baltimore, "The average physician wastes fifty to sixty per cent of his time in going from place to place or in the repetition of uninstructive details of practice." [93] Iris Noble, in her biography for young readers, imagines that as a medical student Osler kept a time diary to determine how he might be more efficient:

> He picked up a paper and pencil lying by the side of the bed. He would write down every minute of that day that he had spent fruitlessly worrying over something that was past or day-dreaming about the future.
>
> When he had completed the list he was appalled. Ten minutes wondering what the professor was thinking because he had been late! At least an hour worrying about an examination that was coming up! Another fifteen minutes after lunch when he and a fellow student had talked aimlessly about what kind of doctors they were going to be when they graduated. . . . It was unbelievable. Yet the record was there. He would have said he had worked hard that day, but instead he had let precious time dribble away through his fingers.[94]

Fictitious or not, Noble depicted the usefulness of keeping such a diary, as many experts now advise. At the end of each day, we should take 10 to 20 minutes to sort out how we spent our time, to see where we might improve, and to reinforce our goals. This exercise can save hours—or even years![95]

Osler knew quite well that such self-discipline is unnatural. As he told students:

> Do not underestimate the difficulty you will have in wringing from your reluctant selves the stern determination to exact the uttermost minute on your schedule. Do not get too interested in one study at the expense of another, but so map out your day that due allowance is given to each. Only in this way can the average student get the best that he can out of his capacities. And it is worth all the pains

and trouble he can possibly take for the ultimate gain—if he can reach his doctorate with system so ingrained that it has become an integral part of his being.[96]

Thayer asked a question that occurred to many: "Wherein lay the secret of his power? What was the manner of the man?" [97] Thayer answered his own question: "His power to hold the mastery of his time was remarkable." [98] Another contemporary remarked, "One had to be in the presence of his conversation but a short time in order to understand his capacity for organization and efficient work. The industry of his heart and hands was soon made apparent." [99] Yet Osler made it look easy. He did not seem overly preoccupied with his own time, at least in the presence of others. He often said that a directing principle of his life was a line from Shakespeare's *Macbeth*: "The flighty purpose never is o'er took / Unless the deed go with it." [100] In a similar vein, J. M. T. Finney observed that " 'Sufficient unto the day is the evil thereof' was the text from which he preached many an effective sermon." [101]A Philadelphia colleague captured the essence of Osler's greatness: his ability to manage the little things in life in such a way that the big things seemed to come about almost effortlessly:

> He had a trait that so many of us lack—greatness in little things— method, system, punctuality, order, the economical use of time. These have been the handmaids to his greater gifts. These have enabled him to widen his usefulness to lands beyond the seas.
> *Seest thou a man diligent in his business? He shall stand before kings.*[102]

In the last year of his life, Osler went to London to see a remarkable woman who was dying from cancer. She had translated from Sanskrit a poem said to have been written around A.D. 400 by an Indian dramatist named Kalidassa. Osler made known his request that the poem be added to any future printing of his essay, "A Way of Life." [103] Posthumously, his wish was honored. The poem reads in part:

> Listen to the Exhortation of the Dawn!
> Look to this Day!
> For it is Life, the very Life of Life.
> · · · · · · · · · · · · · · · · · · ·

For Yesterday is but a Dream
And Tomorrow is only a Vision;
But Today well lived makes
Every Yesterday a Dream of Happiness,
And every Tomorrow a Vision of Hope.
Look well therefore to this Day!
Such is the Salutation of the Dawn!

This was indeed Osler's philosophy of life in day-tight compart-ments.

2

FIND

A

CALLING

Being True to Certain Ideals

William Osler's triumphant journey through life can be understood in at least two complementary ways. On the one hand, he exemplifies the universal hero-myth as elucidated by mythologist Joseph Campbell (Figure 2.1). Summoned by a strange personage, the would-be hero leaves his hut or castle for an unknown realm, encounters a series of tests and helpers under the watchful eye of a shadow presence, and prevailing, brings back to society an elixir that restores something that it had lost. Sir Thomas Browne was Osler's shadow presence, medicine his adventure, and the single-handed writing of a textbook his supreme ordeal. The textbook completed, he gave society a reconciliation of the old humanities with the emerging new medical science. Understood in this

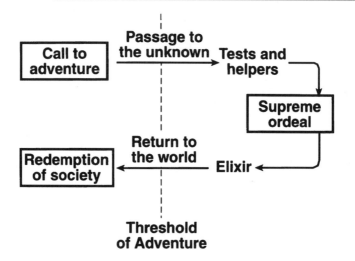

Figure 2.1. The universal hero-myth. (Adapted from Campbell, 1968).

way, Osler's life illustrates the lesson that, as Campbell put it, each of us "shares the supreme ordeal—carries the cross of the re-deemer—not in the bright moments of his tribe's great victories but in the silences of his personal despair." [1]

A more prosaic but perhaps more useful way to understand Osler's journey comes through research into what has been called the adult life cycle. Each of us must deal with age-specific devel-opmental tasks. Today's understanding of adult development began with the work of Carl Jung, with impetus from Erik Erikson, who identified three stages: the stage of identity (from 21 to 35), the stage of generativity (from 35 to 55), and the stage of consolidation (after 55). More recently, psychologist Daniel J. Levinson and his colleagues suggested that we alternate between structure-building and structure-changing periods. Their most striking finding was the relatively low variability of the ages at which each period begins and ends.[2] From this perspective, Osler's life provides a model of healthy adult development.

The third decade of life, the twenties, poses contradictory challenges. The young adult must attempt to establish a stable life structure while simultaneously exploring options and developing a dream. Osler's dream—to become a great clinician and teacher—prompted him to postpone marriage and family for a semimonastic student's life, a solution that is not for everyone. But his life also illustrates that most people have not one but several careers, a phenomenon that is now getting much attention and that bears out the advantage of a liberal education followed by the pursuit of specific skills. Osler found a calling in the deep sense, the matching of his joys and interests to the world's needs, the challenge that his life should contribute to society in a meaningful way. As he told graduating nursing students in 1891:

> Practically, there should be for each of you a busy, useful, and happy life; more you cannot expect; a greater blessing the world cannot bestow. Busy you will certainly be, as the demand is great. . . . Useful your lives must be, as you will care for those who cannot care for themselves. . . . And happy lives shall be yours, because busy and useful; having been initiated into the great secret—that happiness lies in the absorption in some vocation which satisfies the soul; that we are here to add what we can *to*, not to get what we can *from*, life.[3]

EXPLORE THE POSSIBILITIES

Osler, like many young people, made a false start in that he set out toward one vocation and then chose another. He was to be his family's contribution to the Anglican clergy, and to that end he enrolled at Trinity College in Toronto. But the church was rocking from the tremors of Darwinism. People still murmured about the epic 1860 debate that pitted biologist Thomas H. Huxley and the theory of evolution against Bishop Samuel Wilberforce and the literal truth of Genesis. In his first year at Trinity College, Osler became a protégé of Dr. James Bovell, who held the chair of natural theology at Trinity and also taught at Toronto Medical School. Osler began to spend his afternoons at the medical school. In the fall of 1868, he went back to Trinity College for his second year but after a few days announced that he would study medicine instead.

Why did Osler choose medicine? In making this decision, unlike most other major decisions of his life, he agonized before

making up his mind.[4] His most influential teachers, Father W. A.
Johnson and Bovell, stimulated his interest in nature to the extent
that Osler could be called a naturalist. In addition, he no doubt
grasped intuitively that a medical career could bridge the sciences
and the humanities. This, after all, had been a main theme of his
shadow presence, Sir Thomas Browne:

> Thus are there two books from whence I collect my Divinity; besides
> that written one of God, another of his servant Nature, that univer-
> sal and public Manuscript, that lies expans'd unto the eyes of all;
> those that never saw him in the one, have discovered him in the
> other: This was the Scripture and Theology of the Heathens: the
> natural motion of the Sun made them more than admire him, than
> its supernatural station did the Children of Israel.[5]

Of his decision, Osler later wrote: "In the later afternoon Dr.
Bovell would often take me to his lecture at the Toronto School of
Medicine. In this congenial atmosphere what wonder that
Euripides, Aeschylus, Livy, and Horace were dull; conic sections
of trigonometry became an abomination. . . . In October 1868 I
entered the Toronto School of Medicine." [6]

There is no evidence that Osler's decision to study medicine
was couched in high-sounding verbiage, such as the desire to
conquer disease or prevent suffering. He thought medicine would
be fun. As he later advised young people,

> The very first step towards success in any occupation is to become
> interested in it. Locke put this in a very happy way when he said,
> give a pupil "a relish of knowledge" and you put life into his work.
> And there is nothing more certain than that you cannot study well
> if you are not interested in your profession.[7]

Having made this decision, he apparently never questioned its
soundness. In 1899, at 50, he reminisced:

> I started in life—I may as well own up and admit—with just an
> ordinary everyday stock of brains. In my schooldays I was much
> more bent upon mischief than upon books—I say it with regret
> now—but as soon as I got interested in medicine I had only a single
> idea and I do believe that if I have had any measure of success at
> all, it has been solely because of doing the day's work that was
> before me just as faithfully and honestly and energetically as was in
> my power.[8]

Osler brought to his chosen field energy, foresight, and later, uncommon ability to concentrate on each day's tasks.

Although Osler had committed himself to medicine, there was still the issue of what kind of doctor he would be. A generalist or a specialist? A practitioner or a teacher? As it turned out, he pursued a series of roles within medicine: medical student, graduate physician-student, locum tenens for a general practitioner, young faculty member, young professor, active leader of the profession, and finally, elder statesman. He realized that our roles change, that we should stay flexible, and that we should follow our interests and aptitudes. From time to time, he was asked to consider new options. He was tempted by the presidency of a university but turned it down, confiding to a friend that "I am not a suitable man for such a position at all, not having special executive ability." [9] He was urged to run for political office but declined, possibly because he was too prone to see both sides of issues and to seek fairness to everyone concerned.[10] He never lost his basic love of medicine:

> To carefully observe the phenomena of life in all its phases, normal and perverted, to make perfect that most difficult of all arts, the art of observation, to call to aid the science of experimentation, to cultivate the reasoning faculty, so as to be able to know the true from the false—these are our methods. To prevent disease, to relieve suffering and to heal the sick—this is our work. The profession in truth is a sort of guild or brotherhood, any member of which can take up his calling in any part of the world and find brethren whose language and methods and whose aims and ways are identical with his own.[11]

In 1892 he exhorted students at the University of Minnesota:

> Students of Medicine, Apprentices of the Guild, with whom are the promises, and in whom centre our hopes—let me congratulate you on the choice of calling which offers a combination of intellectual and moral interests found in no other profession, and not met with at all in the common pursuits of life—a combination which, in the words of Sir James Paget, "offers the most complete and constant union of those three qualities which have the greatest charm for pure and active minds—novelty, utility, and charity." [12]

While extolling the benefits of a medical career, he was not deaf to rumors of an imminent doctor surplus. Thus in 1894 he reacted to what people were saying at that time:

> But a shrewd old fellow remarked to me the other day, "Yes, many diseases are less frequent, others have disappeared, but new ones are always cropping up, and I notice that with it all there is not only no decrease, but a very great increase in the number of doctors." [13]

In 1897 he said:

> I have heard the fear expressed that in this country the sphere of the physician proper is becoming more and more restricted, and perhaps this is true; but I maintain (and I hope to convince you) that the opportunities are still great, that the harvest truly is plenteous, and the labourers scarcely sufficient to meet the demand.[14]

Although Osler held that there were lots of opportunities in medicine, he also felt that young physicians should explore the possibilities open to them. He told young people to travel, hinting that youth should try to find the best that the world had to offer. And for established physicians, he suggested a "quinquennial brain-dusting"; they should go abroad in search of new ideas. He advised, "Permanence of residence, good undoubtedly for the pocket, is not always best for wide mental vision in the physician." [15] Thus in 1890 he went abroad himself and in "Letters to my House Physicians" told his residents in Baltimore what the opportunities in Europe were like. For example:

> Here in Bern we found a model hospital on the pavilion plan. . . . The Pathological Institute is a large, separate building, with every possible convenience for teaching and research. . . . Bern is one of the Swiss schools most frequented by women, of whom about fifty are at present in attendance. I was told by one of the professors that they were good students.[16]

Osler saw good in every nationality that he studied. Thus he praised the Dutch for having introduced bedside teaching, acknowledging them as "our masters in this as in nearly all the advances in modern civilisation." [17] He congratulated the Danes for "the series of distinguished men who have graced the profession of that country in the past three hundred years." [18] The great French teachers of the early nineteenth century imparted to a generation of American students "enthusiasm, faith in the future, faith in the profession of their choice, accurate methods, and a loyal love of truth." [19] Osler told young physicians that even if they were unable to travel, they could still learn from international colleagues: "Next to a personal knowledge of men, a knowledge of the literature of the profession of different countries will do much to counteract intolerance and Chauvinism." [20]

Osler likewise saw medicine as a life-long adventure. He became a strenuous advocate of continuing education:

> In no single relation of life does the general practitioner show a more illiberal spirit than in the treatment of himself. I do not refer so much to careless habits of living, to lack of routine in work, or to failure to pay due attention to the business side of the profession—sins which so easily beset him—but I would speak of his failure to realize *first*, the need of a lifelong progressive personal training, and *secondly*, the danger lest in the stress of practice he sacrifice that most precious of all possessions, his mental independence. Medicine is a most difficult art to acquire. All the college can do is to teach the student principles, based on facts in science, and give him good methods of work. These simply start him in the right direction, they do not make him a good practitioner—that is his own affair. [21]

Speaking to London medical students in 1907, he used the religious term "calling":

> You are in this profession as a calling, not as a business; as a calling which exacts from you at every turn self-sacrifice, devotion, love and tenderness to your fellow-men. Once you get down to a purely business level, your influence is gone and the true light of your life is dimmed. You must work in the missionary spirit, with a breadth of charity that raises you far above the petty jealousies of life. [22]

In summary, Osler's life and teachings illustrate several desiderata for young people: explore possibilities, learn one's aptitudes, become interested, make choices, keep options open, and—perhaps above all else—find and follow a set of ideals.

BE AN IDEALIST

William Osler came to be in great demand as a speaker at commencement exercises and similar occasions. Rather than meet these obligations with a standard boilerplate address, he honored his audiences with remarks tailored for the occasions. These speeches show "in beautiful but no uncertain terms" his idealism, his reverence for medicine's best traditions and highest standards.[23]

Idealism is commonly defined as thinking or acting according to the way things should be rather than as they are. The pragmatist or realist often sees the idealist as a wishful, falsely optimistic dreamer. Osler encouraged his audiences to be open-eyed but not discouraged by such criticism:

> Nothing in life is more glaring than the contrast between possibilities and actualities, between the ideal and the real. By the ordinary mortal, idealists are regarded as vague dreamers, striving after the impossible; but in the history of the world how often have they gradually moulded to their will conditions the most adverse and hopeless! They alone furnish the *Geist* [spirit] that finally animates the entire body and makes possible reforms and even revolutions. Imponderable, impalpable, more often part of the moral than of the intellectual equipment, are the subtle qualities so hard to define, yet so potent in everyday life, by which these fervent souls keep alive in us the reality of the ideal.[24]

Osler subscribed to what has been called the law of indirect effort, the notion that most rewards and satisfactions come to us in a roundabout way as the result of service to others. Thus he told physicians:

> For better or worse, there are few occupations of a more satisfying character than the practice of medicine, if a man can but once get *orientirt* [oriented; focused] and bring to it the philosophy of honest work, the philosophy which insists that we are here, not to get all we can out of the life about us, but to see how much we can add to it.[25]

He stated this principle even more clearly in his eulogy to Dr. Edward Livingston Trudeau, whose own affliction with tuberculosis prompted his campaign against the disease:

> How true sometimes is the paradox of the Gospel that to save his life a man must lose it! Out of the depths—"from our desolation only may the better life begin". . . . Now and then men are fortunate enough to overcome the worst foes encountered in the battle

of life—chronic ill health, and an enforced residence in a paralyzing environment.[26]

Osler advocated a life of service similar to that endorsed by most great spiritual leaders and counter to the conventional wisdom that life consists mainly of competition, which he saw as especially damaging to scientific work:

> Another unpleasant manifestation of collegiate Chauvinism is the outcome, perhaps, of the very keen competition which at present exists in scientific circles. Instead of a generous appreciation of the work done in other places, there is a settled hostility and a narrowness of judgment but little in keeping with the true spirit of science.[27]

He also recognized that professions are not static, that changing circumstances mandate that we adjust. But, as in a 1903 address to the New Haven Medical Association, he held that the best security in times of rapid change is adherence to basic principles and ideals:

> The times have changed, conditions of practice have altered and are altering rapidly, but when such a celebration takes us back to your origin in simpler days and ways, we find that the ideals which inspired them are ours to-day—ideals which are ever old, yet always fresh and new, and we can truly say in Kipling's words:
>
> > The men bulk big on the old trail,
> >   our own trail, the out trail,
> > They're God's own guides on the Long Trail,
> >   the trail that is always new.[28]

Realizing that idealism requires sacrifice, Osler may have been comforted by the observation of Sir Thomas Browne that "there is no road or ready way to virtue. . . . To perfect virtue, as to Religion, there is required a Panoply, or complete armor." [29]

Osler held that idealism and persistence can bring spectacular achievement even in circumstances that most people would find discouraging. A favorite illustration was the life of William Beaumont, a surgeon in the United States Army who found himself stationed at Fort Mackinac, an obscure outpost between Lake Michigan and Lake Huron. On June 6, 1822, Beaumont was called to treat a young French Canadian named Alexis St. Martin

who was wounded in the abdomen when a shotgun accidentally
went off in a company store. St. Martin survived but was left with
a hole in the stomach—a fistula or abnormal passage between the
stomach and the abdominal wall. Beaumont took advantage of the
unusual complication to study the digestive process as it had never
been studied before. Over many years and thousands of miles, he
continued his experiments on an often reluctant patient. Beaumont emerged as the leading American physiologist of his era. In
his essay "A Backwood Physiologist," Osler observed:

> His work remains a model of patient, persevering investigation, ex-
> periment, and research, and the highest praise we can give him is to
> say that he lived up to and fulfilled the ideals with which he set out,
> and which he expressed when he said: "Truth, like beauty, is 'when
> unadorned, adorned the most,' and in prosecuting these experiments
> and inquiries, I believe I have been guided by its light." [30]

Osler thus attributed Beaumont's greatness largely to idealism and
persistence.

To be sure, Osler's idealism reflected an ebullience about the
long-term benefits of science for humanity more typical of his
period—often called the Progressive Era—than our own. Such
high confidence in science has since been sullied by such phenomena as nuclear weapons, widespread environmental pollution, and
rampant overpopulation. He wrote in a biographical sketch of
Louis Pasteur:

> The future belongs to science. More and more she will control the
> destinies of the nations. Already she has them in her crucible and
> on her balances. In her new mission to humanity she preaches a
> new gospel.[31]

He tried hard to be an optimist even during World War I as he
watched the youth of Britain, including his son, prepare for the
carnage in the trenches of France. Even in that despair, as he
wrote Professor Josiah Royce of Harvard, there was a glimmer of
hope:

> It's the deuce of a mess, this old humanity has got into. We will
> never be any different. I don't suppose we are a bit better than the
> Greeks—in some ways not so good. My chief comfort is to think
> that after all we are living in the childhood of civilization.[32]

And the next year, as the war raged on, he was able to conclude in an address entitled "Science and War":

> And what shall be our final judgement—for or against science? War is more terrible, more devastating, more brutal in its butchery, and the organization of the forces of nature has enabled man to wage it on a titanic scale. . . . To humanity in the gross, science seems a monster, but on the other side is a great credit balance—the enormous number spared the misery of sickness, the unspeakable tortures saved by anaesthesia, the more prompt care of the wounded, the better surgical technique, the lessened time in convalescence, the whole organization of nursing; the wounded soldier would throw his sword into the scale of science—and he is right.[33]

Osler was not naive to the tainted motives of individuals, groups, and nations. But he sought the best in people, saw medicine as much more than a way to make a living, and was himself—to the end—an idealist.

SEE THE BIG PICTURE

Osler realized early in his career that he needed a larger perspective than could be had in Montreal and Canada. The urge to travel came naturally for, as biographer W. R. Bett observed, Osler was "a peripatetic by descent, by upbringing, and by inclination, and a long family association with Cornwall, where many of its members were working as shipbuilders and merchants, instilled in him a love of the sea and a keenness for travelling in foreign lands." [34] After completing his education at Montreal, he went abroad and studied in London, Berlin, Paris, and Vienna, seeking out the medical giants everywhere he went. In Berlin, he observed the famous pathologist Rudolph Virchow and determined to become a great teacher himself.[35] Travel had opened Osler's vista of what he might become and how he might contribute to society.

Although Osler knew what he wanted after that first trip to Europe, he held fast to the notion that one must constantly look elsewhere for fresh perspectives. He maintained:

> The true student is a citizen of the world, the allegiance of whose soul . . . is too precious to be restricted to a single country. The great minds, the great works transcend all limitations of time, of language,

and of race, and the scholar can never feel initiated into the company of the elect until he can approach all of life's problems from the cosmopolitan standpoint. I care not in what subject he may work, the full knowledge cannot be reached without drawing on supplies from other lands than his own—French, English, German, American, Japanese, Russian, Italian—there must be no discrimination by the loyal student, who should willingly draw from any and every source with an open mind and a stern resolve to render unto all their dues.[36]

Travel was considered important not only to learn about one's field but also to learn about humanity:

The strength of a student of men is to travel—to study men, their habits, character, mode of life, their behaviour under varied conditions, their vices, virtues, and peculiarities.[37]

Osler saw medicine as a uniquely global enterprise:

Medicine is the only world-wide profession, following everywhere the same methods, actuated by the same ambitions, and pursuing the same ends. This homogeneity, its most characteristic feature, is not shared by the law, and not by the Church, certainly not in the same degree.[38]

He held that the unity of medicine might be of singular usefulness for the future of humankind:

Linked together by the strong bonds of community of interests, the profession of medicine forms a remarkable world-unit in the progressive evolution of which there is a fuller hope for humanity than in any other direction.[39]

However, he recognized that the greatest threat to such potential unity was chauvinism—unreasonable devotion to or fanaticism about race, sex, time, place, or any other uniqueness. He wrote:

Nationalism has been the great curse of humanity. In no other shape has the Demon of Ignorance assumed more hideous proportions; to no other obsession do we yield ourselves more readily.[40]

Even if young physicians could not afford to travel abroad, they should attempt to find out how things were done elsewhere:

I am not heedless of the truth of the sharp taunt—
How much the fool that hath been sent to Rome,
Exceeds the fool that hath been kept at home.

At any rate, whether he goes abroad or not, let him early escape from the besetting sin of the young physician, *Chauvinism*, that intolerant attitude of mind, which brooks no regard for anything outside his own circle and his own school.[41]

Osler believed that physicians have the opportunity for solidarity not just because of a common enemy—disease—but also because of common methods:

> Of no other profession is the word universal applicable in the same sense. The celebrated phrase used of the Catholic Church is in truth much more appropriate when applied in medicine. It is not the prevalence of disease or the existence everywhere of special groups of men to treat it that betokens this solidarity, but it is the identity throughout the civilized world of our ambitions, our methods and our work.[42]

He could express an almost naive optimism that such solidarity among physicians might someday spread to the rest of society:

> Free, cosmopolitan, no longer hampered by the dogmas of schools, we may feel a just pride in a profession almost totally emancipated from the bondage of error and prejudice. Distinctions of race, nationality, colour, and creed are unknown within the portals of the temple of Æsculapius. Dare we dream that this harmony and cohesion so rapidly developing in medicine, obliterating the strongest lines of division, knowing no tie of loyalty, but loyalty to truth—dare we hope, I say, that in the wider range of human affairs a similar solidarity may ultimately be reached?[43]

Given Osler's cosmopolitan outlook, it is not surprising that three nations—Canada, the United States, and Great Britain—claimed him as their own. And Osler's broad worldview opened up possibilities for his students. As one put it, "The more we learned, the more wonderful his boundless knowledge seemed; the wider our vision, the more limitless his appeared." [44]

The issue of specialism versus generalism recurs in medicine as in other fields, and it evoked controversy in Osler's time as it does today. He was ambivalent. On the one hand he felt that specialization threatened medicine's solidarity. On the other, he

acknowledged that specialization promotes skilled patient care and
scientific progress:

> The restriction of the energies of trained students to narrow fields
> in science, while not without its faults, has been the most important
> single factor in the remarkable expansion of our knowledge. Against
> the disadvantages in a loss of breadth and harmony there is the
> compensatory benefit of a greater accuracy in the application of
> knowledge in specialism, as is well illustrated in the cultivation of
> special branches of practice.[45]

He was concerned that the rising number of specialists would
jeopardize the viabilty of family physicians. But his overarching
concern was that physicians see themselves as parts of an organic
whole working for the common good:

> Members of a corporate body, successful life will depend upon the
> permeation by harmonics which correlate and control the func-
> tions. Isolation means organic inadequacy—each must work in
> sympathy and in union with the other and all for the benefit of the
> community—all toward what Bacon calls the lawful goal of the
> sciences, that human life be endowed with new discoveries and
> power.[46]

Osler believed that to see the big picture, one must have a solid
sense of continuity with the past.

KNOW THE HISTORY

Osler was an outstanding amateur medical historian. The great
pathologist William H. Welch predicted that Osler's "fame as a
serious and scholarly student of medical history and as a bibliog-
rapher" would be only "second to his repute as a great clinical
teacher." [47] Appreciating history helps us transcend the limitations
of a self-serving philosophy:

> In the continual remembrance of a glorious past individuals and
> nations find their noblest inspiration, and if to-day this inspiration,
> so valuable for its own sake, so important in its associations, is
> weakened, is it not because in the strong dominance of the individ-
> ual, so characteristic of a democracy, we have lost the sense of
> continuity?[48]

Osler wrote numerous biographical sketches of great physicians.[49] He believed that biography is the most important component of history:

> History is simply the biography of the mind of man; and our interest in history, and its educational value to us, is directly proportionate to the completeness of our study of the individuals through whom this mind has been manifested.[50]

We should try to understand great figures in the context of their times:

> To understand the old writers one must see as they saw, feel as they felt, believe as they believed—and this is hard, indeed impossible! We may get near them by asking the Spirit of the Age in which they lived to enter in and dwell with us, but it does not always come. . . . Each generation has its own problems to face, looks at truth from a special focus and does not see quite the same outlines as any other.[51]

In addition to biography, he taught the value of understanding the broad sweep of medical history and the roles different peoples had played. For instance, he valued the Hebrew tradition:

> In the medical profession the Jews had a long and honourable record, and among no people is all that is best in our science and art more warmly appreciated; none in the community take more to heart the admonition of the son of Sirach [author of the apocryphal book of Ecclesiasticus]—"Give place to the physician, let him not go from thee, for thou hast need of him." [52]

He valued the ancient Egyptians, acknowledging Imhotep as "the first figure of a physician to stand out clearly from the mists of antiquity," and that "we must come to the land of the Nile for the origin of many of man's most distinctive and highly cherished beliefs." [53] But like most historians of Western civilization, he regarded Greek medicine as the turning point in the evolution of medical science:

> The Greek spirit was the leaven of the old world, the working of which no nationality could resist; thrice it saved western civilisa-

tion, for it had the magic power of . . . making even captive conquerors the missionaries of her culture.[54]

Although he felt that Hippocrates did for medicine what Socrates and Plato did for philosophy, he believed it was erroneous to call Hippocrates the father of medicine in a strict sense:

> From the writings of Plato we may gather many details about the status of physicians in his time. It is very evident that the profession was far advanced and had been progressively developing for a long period before Hippocrates, whom we erroneously, yet with a certain propriety, call the *Father of Medicine*.[55]

Yet he acknowledged the critical importance of the Hippocratic school for developing medical science steeped in empiric observation:

> The critical sense and sceptical attitude of the Hippocratic school laid the foundations of modern medicine on broad lines, and we owe to it: *first*, the emancipation of medicine from the shackles of priestcraft and of caste; *secondly*, the conception of medicine as an art based on accurate observation, and as a science, an integral part of the science of man and of nature; *thirdly*, the high moral ideals, expressed in . . . the Hippocratic oath; and *fourthly*, the conception and realization of medicine as the profession of a cultivated gentleman.[56]

Progress in medicine had, however, been slow until the eighteenth century:

> There have been three great conceptions of the nature of disease. For long centuries it was believed to be the direct outcome of sin. . . . From Hippocrates to Hunter the treatment of disease was one long traffic in hypotheses. . . . In the past fifty years . . . our conception of the nature of disease has been revolutionised.[57]

Osler recognized the importance of appreciating one's own place in history. Where have we come from, and where are we going? Looking back over the nineteenth century, he noted:

> The three great advances of the century have been a knowledge of the mode of controlling epidemic diseases, the introduction of anæsthetics, and the adoption of antiseptic methods in surgery. Beside them all others sink into insignificance, as these three contribute so enormously to the personal comfort of the individual.[58]

More specifically, the nineteenth century had seen the rise of scientific medicine, specialization, and preventive medicine, the appearance of bacteriology, and the advancement of medical education through new schools.[59] He viewed the maturation of twentieth-century medicine with ebullient optimism.

In 1913 Osler made his last visit to the United States. A major purpose was to give a series of lectures in medical history at Yale. Known as the Silliman Lectures and published after Osler's death as *The Evolution of Modern Medicine*, the lectures gave a concise, well-illustrated overview of the entire field. This history still makes good reading, but Osler was at his best during informal discussions of the subject. Three decades later, people could "still remember the enthusiasm of Dr. Osler in his presentation of rare old historical medical subjects or in the enlightening discussion that he gave following someone else's paper." [60]

Osler saw history and tradition as unifying forces opposed to provincialism and special interests:

> With our History, Traditions, Achievements, and Hopes, there is little room for Chauvinism in medicine. The open mind, the free spirit of science, the ready acceptance of the best from any and every source, the attitude of rational receptiveness rather than of antagonism to new ideas, the liberal and friendly relationship between different nations and different sections of the same nation, the brotherly feeling which should characterize members of the oldest, most beneficent and universal guild that the race has evolved in its upward progress—these should neutralize the tendencies upon which I have so lightly touched.[61]

And because medicine is a "universal guild," no nation can make special claims to preeminence—at least over the long haul. Many nations in Western Europe had claimed such preeminence, only to have it taken from them in the next generation. On one occasion Osler wrote, "Minerva Medica is a fickle goddess." [62] On another he explained more fully that

> Minerva Medica has never had her chief temples in any one country for more than a generation or two. For a long period at the Renaissance she dwelt in northern Italy, and from all parts of the world men flocked to Padua and to Bologna. Then for some reason of her own she went to Holland.[63]

After the period of Dutch superiority, the meccas for medical education shifted, in the eighteenth century, to England and Scotland. In the early nineteenth century, Paris became the place to go. Later, German medicine gained ascendancy. It was perhaps because of his due appreciation of such centers of excellence that on his first trip abroad Osler divided his time among Great Britain, France, Germany, and Austria. In an address entitled "The Old and the New," he stressed that we can see future possibilities only within the context of the past:

> The secret of success in an institution . . . is to blend the old with the new, the past with the present in due proportion, and it is not difficult if we follow Emerson's counsel: "We cannot overstate," he says, "our debt to the past, but the moment has the supreme claim; the sole terms on which the past can become ours are its subordination to the present." [64]

JOIN THE ORGANIZATIONS

Osler has been called an organization man.[65] He understood that organizations impart a sense of belonging and connectedness, promote friendships, and counter self-centeredness and contentiousness. He understood that getting involved in organizations, volunteering especially for tasks that others would just as soon avoid, usually pays large long-term dividends that assume many forms: reputation for good work, high profile among people with influence, and reinforcement of personal ideals. Joining and serving organizations is an important example of the law of indirect effort.

By age 32, Osler was "with regularity among those present" at local, regional, and national medical meetings.[66] He became secretary of the Canadian Medical Association. Most people would shun such a time-consuming chore, but it was through the position that Osler got to know leading physicians throughout Canada. Henry Hurd recalled that in this capacity Osler

> encountered many difficulties in the way of personal feeling and local prejudice on the part of the physicians. Difficulties were smoothed over and asperities were softened by his courtesy, good humour, and above all, by his ever present and sparkling wit. At one

time, however, it became necessary for him to administer a speedy rebuke to a wrong-headed, obstinate and somewhat unmanageable person, which was done so effectively as to prevent any further difficulties from that source during the remainder of the meeting.[67]

Such was Osler's influence that, when he moved to the United States at age 35, he was made president-elect of the Canadian Medical Association. In this position he did "more than any other member of our profession to bring about cordial and intimate relationships between its members in the United States and Canada." [68]

Besides supporting existing organizations, Osler started new ones. Thus in Baltimore, "the Medical Society, the Journal Club, the Historical Club, and other associations, were organized in quick succession." [69] In 1900 he founded a Laennec Society—possibly the first organization in the world solely dedicated to the study of tuberculosis.[70] Later, in England, he patterned the Association of Physicians of Great Britain and Ireland after those he had been associated with in the United States.[71] Osler saw organizations as a way to bring people together to promote goodwill, common interests, and service to society.

Despite his own commitment, Osler knew that many people protested that organization work only wasted their time. He was "very scrupulous" about attending meetings even when he didn't feel like going. When a student confided his reluctance to go to the local medical society meeting because he was unsure whether he would get anything out of it, Osler responded, "Do you think I go for what I can get out of it or for what I can put into it?" Hurd observed that those who knew Osler "felt a deep impression that in all activities in medical societies and in behalf of his students he labored solely to inspire them with a love of work for its own sake and for what he felt to be its final effect upon their growth and development." [72] Osler also knew that many people refused to participate in organizations because they found something objectionable about them. Again his own best example, he strenuously objected to the examination system imposed by London's Royal College of Physicians but nevertheless made time to serve on its council and Library Committee.[73] He knew that organizations, like people, must be accepted as we find them.

Osler considered such participation to be a duty, stating that

> no physician has a right to consider himself as belonging to himself;
> but all ought to regard themselves as belonging to the profession,
> inasmuch as each is a part of the profession; and care for the part
> naturally looks to care for the whole.[74]

Cushing's biography mentions no fewer than 110 associations and
societies in which Osler participated at various times. Of these, 45
were American, 43 British, 13 Canadian, 5 international, and 4
French.[75] Although Osler was not a dues-paying member of all of
these organizations, he participated whenever he could. Lewellys
F. Barker marveled at Osler's ability to exert influence through his
self-control and character, noting that Osler

> grasped, as it were intuitively, the newer principles of association
> and of group organization. A man of many selves, he could enter
> into helpful association with many different groups, letting his mind
> interact with the other minds of each group for the purpose of
> arriving at ideas, feelings and impulses in common. More than most
> he had learned how to live with other men, to discuss without
> antagonism, to secure co-operation by the subtle psychic process of
> reciprocal penetration. In this lay the secret of his co-ordinating
> power.[76]

Osler's career illustrates that service in voluntary organizations
fosters the development of leadership and management skills necessary for career advancement. He absorbed such skills through
voluntary medical organizations and later used them to organize
medical clinics. He held that medical societies had several functions:

> No class of men need friction so much as physicians; no class gets
> less. The daily round of a busy practitioner tends to develop an
> egoism of a most intense kind, to which there is no antidote. The
> few set-backs are forgotten. The mistakes are often buried, and ten
> years of successful work tends to make a man touchy, dogmatic,
> intolerant of correction and abominably self-centered. To this men-
> tal attitude the medical society is the best corrective, and a man
> misses a good part of his education who does not get knocked about
> a bit by his colleagues in discussions and criticisms.[77]

He urged participation not only to further education but also to
promote fellowship:

> By no means the smallest advantage [of medical societies] is the
> promotion of harmony and good-fellowship. Medical men, particu-
> larly in smaller places, live too much apart and do not see enough
> of each other. In large cities, we rub each other's angles down and
> carom off each other without feeling the shock very much, but it is
> an unfortunate circumstance that in many towns the friction, being
> on a small surface, hurts; and mutual misunderstandings arise to
> the destruction of all harmony.[78]

Such involvement was not just desirable; it was necessary:

> You cannot afford to stand aloof from your professional colleagues
> in any place. Join their associations, mingle in their meetings, give
> the best of your talents, gathering here, scattering there; but every-
> where showing that you are at all times faithful students, as willing
> to teach as to be taught. Shun as most pernicious that frame of
> mind, too often, I fear, seen in physicians, which assumes an air of
> superiority and limits as worthy of your communion only those with
> satisfactory collegiate or sartorial credentials. The passports of your
> fellowship should be honesty of purpose, and a devotion to the
> highest interests of our profession, and these you will find widely
> diffused, sometimes apparent only when you get beneath the crust
> of a rough exterior.[79]

Osler's involvement in medical societies led to an ever-widening
sphere of influence as he moved from a student's society to county,
national, and finally international organizations. He recognized
that it was through organizations that physicians were in the best
position to pool their resources to promote good medicine and
public health. However, he also recognized that the numerous
organizations in medicine tended to fragment the profession:

> So vast . . . and composite has the profession become, that the
> physiological separation, in which dependent parts are fitly joined
> together, tends to become pathological, and while some parts suffer
> necrosis and degeneration, others, passing the normal limits, be-
> come disfiguring and dangerous outgrowths on the body medical.
> The dangers and evils which threaten harmony among the units, are
> internal, not external. And yet, in it more than in any other profes-
> sion . . . is complete organic unity possible.[80]

Although Osler preached professional solidarity, he was not blind
to quarrels and divisions. Disagreements among doctors often
exploded into feuds that became public knowledge and split com-

munities. Speaking to the New Haven Medical Association in 1903, he said:

> The first, and in some respects the most important, function is that mentioned by the wise founders of your parent society—to lay a foundation for that unity and friendship which is essential to the dignity and usefulness of the profession. Unity and friendship! How we all long for them, but how difficult to attain! Strife seems rather to be the very life of the practitioner, whose warfare is incessant against disease and against ignorance and prejudice, and, sad to have to admit, he too often lets his angry passions rise against his professional brother. The quarrels of doctors make a pretty chapter in the history of medicine. Each generation seems to have had its own.

He went on to review how even from ancient times, the medical profession had been divided by such quarrels:

> The Coans and the Cnidians, the Arabians and the Galenists, the humoralists and the solidists, the Brunonians and the Broussaisians, the homœpaths and the regulars, have, in different centuries, rent the robe of Æsculapius. But these larger quarrels are becoming less and less intense, and in the last century no new one of moment sprang up, while it is easy to predict that in the present century, when science has fully leavened the dough of homœpathy, the great breach of our day will be healed. But in too many towns and smaller communities miserable frictions prevail, and bickerings and jealousies mar the dignity and usefulness of the profession.[81]

But looking beyond such "miserable frictions," he found an enormous amount of goodwill in what he called a "community of interests" dedicated to raising the standards of his profession:

> One of the most gratifying features of our professional life is the good feeling which prevails between the various sections of the country. I do not see how it could be otherwise. One has only to visit different parts and mingle with the men to appreciate that everywhere good work is being done, everywhere an earnest desire to elevate the standard of education, and everywhere the same self-sacrificing devotion on the part of the general practitioner. Men will tell you that commercialism is rife, that the charlatan and the humbug were never so much in evidence, and that in our ethical standards there has been a steady declension. These are the Elijahs who are always ready to pour out their complaints, mourning that they are not better than their fathers. Few men have had more

favourable opportunities than I have had to gauge the actual conditions in professional private life, in the schools, and in the medical
societies, and . . . I am filled with thankfulness for the present
and with hope for the future.[82]

Osler acknowledged that each generation will have its prophets of
doom but that these should be counterbalanced by those who
maintain the highest professional standards:

In every age there have been Elijahs ready to give up in despair at
the progress of commercialism in the profession. Garth says in 1699
(*Dispensary*)—

Now sickening Physick hangs her pensive head
And what was once a Science, now's a Trade.

Of medicine, many are of the opinion . . . that the ancients had
endeavoured to make it a science and failed, and the moderns to
make it a trade and have succeeded. To-day the cry is louder than
ever, and in truth there are grounds for alarm; but on the other
hand, we can say to these Elijahs that there are more than 7,000
left who have not bowed the knee to this Baal.[83]

He thus believed that organizations help their members take the
high road in the conviction that what benefits society, in the long
run benefits their profession and themselves.

LEAVE A LEGACY

The four basic human needs, according to Stephen R. Covey and
his colleagues, are to live, to love, to learn, and to leave a legacy.[84]
Like most people, Osler began to dwell increasingly on his legacy
as he got older. At 48 he told Maryland physicians that "to carry
on, though dead, the work he was interested in while living, is the
nearest approach a man can make to cheating the great enemy." [85]
Osler recognized that our main legacy to those we leave behind
should be a better, safer world. He acknowledged the dark side of
human nature but was optimistic that "the leaven of science,
working in the individual" could improve humanity's prognosis:

Who runs may read the scroll which reason has placed as a warning
over the human menageries: "chained, not tamed." And yet who can

doubt that the leaven of science, working in the individual, leavens in some slight degree the whole social fabric. Reason is at least free, or nearly so; the shackles of dogma have been removed, and faith herself, freed from a morganatic alliance [that is, an alliance between the noble and the common], finds in the release great gain.[86]

Osler's legacy can be divided into at least five areas. First was his work toward elevating the standards of medicine. In the late nineteenth century there were many medical schools of doubtful quality, and rigorous licensing of physicians by state boards was almost nonexistent. Advocating higher standards for physicians, he was a major proponent for the creation of such a state board in Maryland:

> To move surely we must move slowly, but firmly and fearlessly, confident in the justness of our claims on behalf of the profession and of the public, and animated solely with a desire to secure to the humblest citizen of this great country in the day of his tribulation and in the hour of his need, a skill worthy of the enlightened humanity which we profess, and of the noble calling in which we have the honor to serve.[87]

He advocated not only better medical education but also universal access to quality health care, at least for urgent problems. He urged physicians and schools to rise above their narrow self-interests and support stricter standards.

A second legacy was his contribution to the medical literature. Many of his articles are still quoted. A third was his promotion of unity and harmony in the medical profession. A fourth legacy came through his abilities as a fund-raiser for worthy causes. As Cushing noted:

> To whatever soil he was transplanted, the same Osler grew and flourished, modifying his environment more than it modified him. It is interesting to see how consistently he began anew in Oxford with precisely the same projects as those which had engaged him in Montreal, Philadelphia, and Baltimore. . . . Lavish in his own name when it came to giving, he must have been a hard man to refuse when in an offhand way he asked for help.[88]

The fifth legacy, the one that occupied Osler during his final years, arose from his love of books and libraries. This passion ultimately produced a special library in his own memory, a haven for scholars—the Osler Library at McGill University.

His interest in libraries came naturally from his commitment to medical and general scholarship. Wherever he moved, the libraries benefited. He supported libraries in Montreal, Philadelphia, Baltimore, and Washington, D.C., and—remarkably—he continued to support each library after he had moved elsewhere.[89] His involvement intensified at Oxford, possibly because he had more leisure time. In 1906 he was made an ex officio curator of the Bodleian Library at Oxford, an appointment meant to be largely honorary. Little had been done for the library for more than four decades. That soon changed. Osler immersed himself in the library's affairs, stimulated the staff, encouraged the acquisition of noteworthy books, and made "constant reference in his brief letters" to the library's progress. After Osler died, the Bodleian officials noted, "We miss him, not because he promoted this or that piece of work, but because of his living influence, which helped and stimulated us all." [90]

Especially during his Oxford period, Osler spent much of his time collecting books with the aim of giving them to libraries either then or through his will. When he charged patients for consultations, he spoke of "sanctifying the fee" through book purchases. While visiting in Rome in 1909, for example, he received a fee for seeing an American patient who happened to be there:

> I sanctified my fee by buying 3 copies of Vesal [Vesalius, the great sixteenth-century anatomist], 2nd edition, fine one for myself, a 1st for McGill (300 fr. was too stiff, but it goes for 500!) & another for the Frick library.[91]

Recognizing that his own passion for books bordered on bibliomania, Osler defended the

> class of men in the profession to whom books are dearer than to teachers or practitioners—a small, a silent band. . . . The profane call them bibliomaniacs, and in truth they are at times irresponsible and do not always know the difference between *meum* [mine] and *tuum* [yours]. . . . Loving books partly for their contents, partly for the sake of the authors, they . . . [help] keep alive the sentiment of historical continuity in the profession. . . . We need more men of this class, particularly in this country, where every one carries in his pocket the tape-measure of utility.[92]

But as his personal library grew, he began to be concerned that it would be dissembled after his death and disposed of unceremoniously.

> When a man devotes his life to some particular branch of study and accumulates, year by year, a more or less complete literature, it is very sad after his death to have such a library come under the hammer—almost the inevitable fate.[93]

While reviewing the collections of the Pepys Library, Osler conceived the idea of preparing an elaborate catalog of his own collection. Partially completed at the time of his death, it was eventually published as the *Bibliotheca Osleriana*—a massive list of 7,783 works illustrating the history of medicine and science, most of which are annotated by Osler himself. Osler arranged that his library would be left, largely intact, to McGill University. He envisioned the fate of his books:

> I like to think of my few books in an alcove of a fire-proof library of some institution that I love; at the end of an alcove an open fireplace and a few easy chairs, and on the mantelpiece an urn with my ashes and my bust or portrait through which my astral self, like the Bishop of St. Praxed's, could peek at the books I have loved and enjoy the delight with which kindred souls still in the flesh would handle them.[94]

And thus, save only for the open fireplace, his library stands today, elegantly housed at McGill, a tribute to Osler's work, priorities, and personality.

Granting that few can match Osler's career success, what legacy is within the reach of most of us? What if we do not have the equivalent of a large and valuable book collection? William Osler made it clear that it suffices to devote our lives to the conscientious pursuit of a higher cause. He made this point strongly in his famous essay "An Alabama Student." The student in question was Dr. John Y. Bassett of Huntsville, Alabama. Reviewing the literature on malaria in the South, Osler came across two reports written by Bassett between 1849 and 1850. Curious to find out what happened to Bassett, he wrote to Huntsville and was referred to Bassett's daughter, who supplied him with a packet of letters that her father had written from Paris in 1836. Bassett, it turned out, had left his family and his secure practice in Huntsville to go to Paris, the medical mecca of that day, to become a better doctor. His letters revealed a highly motivated, deeply committed, and philosophical man who wanted to give his best to the profession. Bassett's life was cut short at age 46 by tuberculosis. Osler ended his essay about Bassett with these consoling words:

> To have striven, to have made an effort, to have been true to certain ideals—this alone is worth the struggle. Now and again in a generation, one or two snatch something from dull oblivion; but for the rest of us, sixty years—we, too, are with Bassett and his teachers, and

> No one asks
> Who or what we have been,
> More than he asks what waves,
> In the moonlit solitudes mild
> Of the midmost ocean, have swelled,
> Foam'd for a moment, and gone.[95]

3

FIND

MENTORS

The Young Person's Friend

Osler attributed his success not only to hard work and career planning but also to a rich network of interpersonal relationships. He recognized that what makes or breaks our luck more often than not is the quality of our bonds with fellow humans. In his formative years, he sought out older people who could offer knowledge, skills, and insights. In his maturity, he sought out younger people who could magnify his effectiveness and ensure his legacy. Such relationships are now taught as *mentoring*, today's buzzword for an ancient concept.

Mentor in Greek legend was the faithful servant and advisor to Ulysses, king of Ithaca. Embarking for the Trojan war, Ulysses left his wife, Penelope, and his son, Telemachus, under Mentor's care. Telemachus absorbed from

Mentor practical wisdom of the kind that cannot be learned from books. Osler showed his familiarity with the story in a 1903 birthday card to his own son, Revere:

> Many happy returns of The Day
> to the small Telemachus
> Care of Mistress
> Penelope
> from old Ulysses
> on the Island of Aegia

Osler identified with Ulysses since he too was often made the absentee father by a sense of duty.[1] The poet Robert Bly, in *Iron John*, argues that the industrial revolution accelerated the need for mentors by removing the father's workplace from his neighborhood, leaving children to fend for themselves. Mentoring has become an urgent societal priority. William Osler's life offers textbook examples of how to go about finding mentors of various types and how to become a mentor in turn.

BEGIN THE JOURNEY

Osler's relationship with his father was not especially close, perhaps because the latter was older and in failing health during the youngest son's formative years. To his credit, Featherstone Osler supported young William's coming under the influence of other men. When it came time for Osler to dedicate his great 1892 textbook, *The Principles and Practice of Medicine*, he chose to honor three of them:

> To
> The Memory of My Teachers:
> WILLIAM ARTHUR JOHNSON
> Priest of the Parish of Weston, Ontario
> JAMES BOVELL
> of the Toronto School of Medicine
> and of the
> University of Trinity College, Toronto
> ROBERT PALMER HOWARD
> Dean of the Medical Faculty and Professor of Medicine
> McGill University, Montreal

Between 1866 and 1871, Osler formed close relationships with Johnson, Bovell, and Howard, each of whom helped broaden his horizons while narrowing his career options. Collectively they launched the young medical graduate on his 1872 trip to the British Isles and Europe, where he would formulate his dream of becoming a great clinical teacher, the dream symbolized by the textbook. The three men were strikingly different.

Osler's introduction to Father Johnson, founder and warden at Trinity College School in Weston, Ontario, was reviewed in the previous chapter. Osler later wrote that Johnson was "a good field botanist, a practical palaeontologist, an ardent microscopist," who "had a rare gift for imparting knowledge and inspiring enthusiasm." [2] Johnson believed that learning to think was more important than memorizing facts. This philosophy, avant-garde as it was during the 1860s, infuriated the school's stern headmaster but delighted young Willie Osler, who quickly fell under Johnson's influence. It was from Johnson that Osler acquired a passion for science.

Johnson was a naturalist in the tradition of priests who studied nature to learn more about God, a discipline known as natural theology. [3] Natural theology flourished during the eighteenth and early-nineteenth centuries and reached its zenith with the 1802 publication of *Natural Theology; or Evidences of the Existence and Attributes of the Deity, Collected from the Appearances of Nature* by William Paley, an English clergyman. Paley's book began with the famous analogy that just as the intricacies of a watch imply the existence of a watchmaker, so do the incredible intricacies of nature imply the existence of a divine creator. It was in this spirit that Johnson became a dedicated amateur naturalist and acquired one of the few microscopes to be found in rural Canada.

Johnson made frequent field trips to obtain specimens for his microscopic studies. Harvey Cushing gave this account of Johnson's enthusiasm:

> Everything interested him, the structure of the hair of different animals from the caribou to the flying squirrel, the structure and growth of wood, the study of fossils and minerals, the finer anatomy of moths and butterflies and insects of every kind, some of which he unblushingly transferred from his own person or bed to the stage of the microscope; seeds and shells, ferns and mosses, bones and

teeth of vertebrates . . . to the molar of an old cow killed on the railway track.[4]

Osler soon succumbed to Johnson's spell, as he later wrote:

> Imagine the delight of a boy of an inquisitive nature to meet a man who cared nothing about words but who knew about things—who knew the stars in their courses and who could tell us their names, who delighted in the woods in springtime, and told us about the frogspawn and the caddis worms, and who read to us in the evenings . . . who showed us with the microscope the marvels in a drop of dirty pond water, and who on Saturday excursions up the river could talk of the Trilobites and the Orthoceratites and explain the formation of the earth's crust. No more dry husks for me after such a diet. . . . From the study of nature to the study of man was an easy step.[5]

Cushing found it "truly amazing" that Johnson could similarly interest a teenaged boy in the writings of Sir Thomas Browne.[6] Under Johnson's tutelage Osler embraced both the natural sciences and the humanities. In many ways, his course was set.

Osler's relationship with Johnson illustrates what might be called the natural method for forming a mentor–protégé relationship. The relationship should not be forced. The would-be mentor must have competence, character, and patience. The would-be protégé must show ability, enthusiasm, and a willingness to help. Their personalities should be compatible. A shared sense of humor is highly desirable, since the relationship should be fun. Osler must have stood out among Johnson's pupils on field trips because of his energy, enthusiasm, and aptitude. Johnson recognized that he had discovered a potential coinvestigator, a person who someday might make independent observations. Osler began to focus his attention on freshwater polyzoa, and in a paper written a decade later, drawn on notebooks he had written as a teenager, referred to Johnson as "my friend":

> In the summer of 1867, during a visit of my friend, the Rev. W. A. Johnson of Weston, I showed him the masses and we agreed to submit them to examination with the microscope, not having any idea of their real nature. Judge of our delight when we found the whole surface of the jelly was composed of a collection of tiny animals of surpassing beauty, each of which thrust out to our view in the zoophyte trough a crescent-shaped crown of tentacles.[7]

Osler's later mentoring relationships followed much the same pattern. The eager young man expressed interest in another's work, formed a bond, and received guidance, focus, and affection.

CULTIVATE TEACHERS

Father Johnson, like all good mentors, realized that there comes a point at which promising protégés must be passed to other hands. Osler's next mentor–protégé relationship sprang from Johnson's own friendship with James Bovell, a Toronto physician. Bovell was an unusual man with a cosmopolitan background. He was born in Barbados and had studied medicine in London, Edinburgh, and Dublin, where he knew such nineteenth century giants as Thomas Addison, Richard Bright, Robert Graves, and William Stokes. He practiced in Barbados for a while but later moved to Canada, where he organized a medical department for Trinity College in Toronto and served as dean and professor of the Institutes of Medicine. He then joined the faculty of the Toronto Medical School but kept the chair of natural theology at Trinity. His infatuation with natural theology led him to Father Johnson's field trips, and it was through this shared interest that Osler came to know him.[8]

Bovell's credentials and breadth of knowledge made a deep impression on Osler. An 1869 entry in one of Osler's student notebooks contains this entry on the flyleaf:

> James Bovell, M.D., M.R.C.P. Prof. Nat. Theology in Trinity College Toronto. Lecturer on Institutes of Medicine, Toronto School of Med. Consulting Physician to Toronto General Hospital. Physician to Lying-in Hospital. Lay Secretary to Provincial Synod. Author of Outline of Natural Theology, &c. &c. &c. James Bovell.[9]

Osler spent the winter of 1869-1870 in Bovell's residence, in payment for which he kept Bovell's appointments and prepared specimens. An unexpected boon was the opportunity to linger in Bovell's library. Osler reminisced nearly 50 years later:

> It has been remarked that for a young man the privilege of browsing in a large and varied library is the best introduction to a general education. My opportunity came in the winter of '69–70. Having sent his family to the West Indies, Dr. Bovell took consulting rooms

in Spadina Avenue not far away from his daughter. . . . He gave
me a bedroom in the house, and my duties were to help to keep
appointments—an impossible job!—and to cut sections and prepare
specimens. Having catholic and extravagant tastes he had filled the
room with a choice and varied collection of books. After a review of
the work of the day came the long evening for browsing, and that
winter [1869–1870] gave me a good first-hand acquaintance with
the original works of many of the great masters.[10]

Bovell thus stirred Osler's interests both in medicine and in literature.

Although Osler admired Bovell, he found flaws that were to be
avoided. Bovell was something of a dilettante. He was sadly im-
practical, hopelessly diffuse in his interests, and lacked punctuality. In an unsigned obituary probably written by Osler, Bovell was
criticized for "a want of that dogged persistency of purpose without
which a great work can scarcely be accomplished." [11] When Osler
confided his desire to make a decent living to a subsequent mentor,
he wrote, "I am sorry to have to appear so mercenary, but the
recollection of my old friend Dr. Bovell, who tried to work at
Physiology and Practice both and failed in both, is too green in my
memory to allow me to take any other course." [12] Osler revered
Bovell almost as a father despite the flaws. In 1903 he told Toronto
medical students:

> To one of my teachers I must pay in passing the tribute of filial
> affection. There are men here to-day who feel as I do about Dr.
> James Bovell—that he was one of those finer spirits, not uncommon
> in life, touched to finer issues only in a suitable environment.[13]

Osler's mentor–protégé relationship with Bovell illustrates that the
best mentors are those who allow us to share their lives to the
extent that we see their shortcomings as well as their strengths.
Bovell stimulated Osler's interest in medicine and literature and
convinced him, indirectly, of the importance of focus, determination, and persistence toward goals.

Although Bovell's return to the West Indies, where he later left
medicine for the clergy, was upsetting to Osler, he soon found a
replacement in Robert Palmer Howard. It was Howard who
pointed him most clearly toward his destiny to become a great
generalist physician. Osler later reminisced:

> When in September, 1870, he [Bovell] wrote to me that he did not
> intend to return from the West Indies I felt I had lost a father and
> a friend; but in Robert Palmer Howard, of Montreal, I found a noble
> step-father, and to these two men, and to my first teacher, the Rev.
> W. A. Johnson, of Weston, I owe my success in life—if success
> means getting what you want and being satisfied with it.[14]

But Osler's mentor–protégé relationship with Howard, unlike his
previous relationships with Johnson and Bovell, did not emerge
from an established friendship. Osler had to seek Howard out, and
the way he went about it illustrates that finding suitable mentors
is usually an active process requiring thought, energy, and a measure of risk taking.

Howard was a tall, rather stern man who seemed almost totally
caught up in medicine. Cushing describes him as "a courtly gentleman, scholarly, industrious, stimulating as a teacher" who,
"though the students of the day felt that he was devoid of humour,"
was "nevertheless popular with them." [15] But most students found
him difficult to approach. Osler succeeded to the extent that he
could report, "The summer of 1871, spent at Montreal, brought
me into almost filial relations with Dr. Palmer Howard, whose
library was at my disposal." [16] Within a year of losing Bovell, Osler
had found another mentor who regarded him almost as a son and
who gave him access to the best medical library in Montreal.

How did Osler succeed where others hardly dared to try?
Tradition holds that he went to Howard's home late one night
seeking to clarify a point Howard had made in a lecture. To do this,
Osler had to overcome fear of rejection, the anxiety known to
salespersons as "call reluctance." Iris Noble conjectured how Osler
must have felt:

> His feet had led him, consciously or unconsciously, to Dr. Howard's
> house. There was a light on in one of the rooms; he could see it.
> But it must be nearly ten o'clock now. Dr. Howard might have gone
> to bed. That light—but no, he didn't dare ring the bell. Dr. Howard
> would be furious with him. Yet what did it matter if he was angry, if
> only he would explain.[17]

Howard did not have a ready answer to Osler's question, and soon
the two men were poring over books.[18] Howard invited Osler to
return. He offered the use of his library. They began to share other
interests, especially pathology. Howard often performed autopsies

on his own patients. Osler became his assistant, helping him prepare specimens. The relationship blossomed.

From Osler's approach to Howard can be gleaned several tips on finding mentors. First, those at the top of their professions are often rather lonely people who are naturally inclined toward younger people whose interest seems genuine. Second, highly successful people usually prefer that requests for their time be short and specific. Third, the risks of approaching such people are seldom as great as we fear. Finally, the potential protégé should have something to offer. Successful people take pride in having discovered a star. Osler knew that his ability and enthusiasm would be useful to the great professor. In 1905 Osler acknowledged the pivotal role that Howard had played in his career:

> In my early days I came under the influence of an ideal student-teacher, the late Palmer Howard, of Montreal. If you ask what manner of man he was, read Matthew Arnold's noble tribute to his father in his well-known poem, *Rugby Chapel*. When young, Dr. Howard had chosen a path—"path to a clear-purposed goal," and he pursued it with unswerving devotion. With him the study and the teaching of medicine were an absorbing passion, the ardour of which neither the incessant and ever-increasing demands upon his time nor the growing years could quench.[19]

Osler internalized Howard's mastery of medicine as a "clear-purposed goal" and his role in life as that of the "ideal student-teacher." Howard delighted in Osler's decision to study medicine under the great masters of Great Britain and Europe. For his part, Osler would say, only partly in jest, "Advice is sought to confirm a position already taken." [20]

Osler's sequential relationships with Johnson, Bovell, and Howard were thus remarkably similar. Each was an educator who entered Osler's life at a propitious time and helped him through a transition. Each relationship lasted in its intense phase no more than two or three years. Each mentor recognized when his own contribution to Osler's development was essentially complete. Each willingly passed the young man along to the next level. Osler's dedication of his textbook to the memory of these teachers acknowledged their silent partnership in his career development.

Although Johnson, Bovell, and Howard were Osler's most conspicuous mentors, there were many others. By his early twenties,

Osler had established a knack for forming friendships with older men who could help him. In Europe, he sought out well-known, influential teachers in a way that was neither contrived nor affected. As Osler later put it, "I have always loved old men." [21] He did not seek out merely the famous and more fortunate. Cushing observed that by age 25 Osler "never failed to ingratiate himself, wherever he might be, with the older practitioners in particular, towards whom he always felt especially drawn." [22] Osler treated his elders as if they were his contemporaries, and "if in the course of conversation a person's years were in question he was wont to reply, 'Oh, he's just our age.' " [23]

HAVE HEROES

Osler's mentors were not limited to people he knew personally. He studied the lives and works of great physicians, writers, and other historical figures with the aim of internalizing their finer qualities. Although something of a hero worshiper, he sought to understand such persons in the context of their times. They formed his reference group, the people with whom he identified and whom he tried to emulate. His major hero was Sir Thomas Browne, whom he called his "lifelong mentor."

Osler called Browne's *Religio Medici* "the most precious book in my library" and told students that

> from such books come subtle influences which give stability to character and help to give a man a sane outlook on the complex problems of life. . . . Mastery of self, conscientious devotion to duty, deep human interest in human beings—these best of all lessons you must learn now or never: and these are some of the lessons which may be gleaned from the writings of Sir Thomas Browne.[24]

On another occasion, he said that there were

> three lessons to be gathered from the life of Sir Thomas Browne, all of them of value to-day. First, we see in him a man who had an ideal education. . . . The second important lesson we may gain is that he presents a remarkable example in the medical profession of a man who mingled the waters of science with the oil of faith. . . .

The third lesson to be drawn is that the perfect life may be led in a very simple, quiet way.[25]

Reviewing his own life at age 70, Osler again acknowledged Browne:

Paraphrasing my lifelong mentor—of course I refer to Sir Thomas Browne—among multiplied acknowledgement I can lift up one hand to heaven that I was born of honest parents, that modesty, humility, patience and veracity lay in the same egg, and came into the world with me. To have had a happy home in which unselfishness reigned, parents whose self-sacrifice remains a blessed memory, brothers and sisters helpful far beyond the usual measure—all these make a picture delightful to look back upon. Then to have had the benediction of friendship follow one like a shadow, to have always had the sense of comradeship in work, without the petty pin-pricks of jealousies and controversies, to be able to rehearse in the sessions of sweet, silent thought the experiences of long years without a single bitter memory—to have and to do all this fills the heart with gratitude.[26]

Although Sir Thomas Browne was Osler's most durable historical mentor, there were many others. With his interest in the broad sweep of Western thought, Osler naturally admired the ancient Greeks. To them he traced the interconnectedness of the sciences and the humanities:

Nature is ever special, and a knowledge of her laws may form a sound Grecian foundation upon which to build the superstructure of a life as useful to the State, and as satisfying to the inner needs of a man, as if the ground-work were classics and literature. The two, indeed, cannot be separated. What naturalist is uninfluenced by Aristotle, what physician worthy of the name, whether he knows it or not, is without the spirit of Hippocrates?[27]

And again:

We are fortunate in having had preserved the writings of the two most famous of the Greek philosophers—the great idealist, Plato, whose "contemplation of all time and all existence" was more searching than that of his predecessors, fuller than that of any of his disciples, and the great realist, Aristotle, to whose memory every department of knowledge still pays homage.[28]

Osler also sought inspiration from the great physicians of the past. Foremost among these were three English physicians, Thomas

Linacre (1450–1524), William Harvey (1578–1657), and Thomas Sydenham (1624–1689). Paneled portraits of these men hung above the fireplace in the library of Osler's home in Baltimore and later at Oxford. Symbolizing different aspects of medicine, Linacre, Harvey, and Sydenham were a historical parallel to the real-life triumvirate of Johnson, Bovell, and Howard.[29]

Thomas Linacre was Osler's model of the medical humanist. Linacre belonged to a small group of fifteenth- and sixteenth-century scholars who restored Greek learning to medicine. He was best known for translating many of the works of Galen, the second-century Greek physician whose theories dominated medicine until the Renaissance, from Greek into Latin. Linacre also taught Erasmus, the great Renaissance scholar and theologian, and was the principal founder of London's College of Physicians. Osler praised Linacre especially for his focus on Greek thought, saying, "Not until Greece rose from the dead did light and liberty come to the human mind, and it is the special glory of Linacre that he became . . . the 'restorer of learning in this country.' "[30] He admired Linacre's literary inclinations:

> Linacre, the type of the literary physician, must ever hold a unique place in the annals of our profession. . . . Painstaking, accurate, critical, hypercritical perhaps, he remains to-day the chief literary representative of British medicine. . . . By the neglect of the study of the humanities, which has been far too general, the profession loses a very precious quality.[31]

Linacre thus combined expertise in medicine with general scholarship, a combination that Osler also modeled, especially during the later years of his life.

William Harvey is perhaps the most famous English physician of all time on account of his discovery of the circulation of the blood. Harvey contradicted an explanation that had been handed down for centuries by followers of Galen, who held that blood ebbed and flowed through invisible pores in the heart muscle. Because Galen was regarded as infallible, Harvey faced violent opposition. In 1906, Osler praised Harvey for his patience:

> Sorely tried as he must have been, and naturally testy, only once in his writings . . . does the old Adam break out. With his temperament, and with such provocation, this is an unexampled record, and one can appreciate how much was resisted in those days when

tongue and pen were free. Over and over again he must have restrained himself. . . . To no man does the right spirit in these matters come by nature, and I would urge upon our younger Fellows and Members . . . to emulate our great exemplar, whose work shed such lustre upon British Medicine, and whom we honour in this college not less for the scientific method which he inculcated than for the admirable virtues of his character.[32]

When Osler was asked to deliver the prestigious Harveian Oration at England's Royal College of Physicians, he found various materials granted to Harvey, such as his Royal Charter, his pension, and his diplomas, all in need of care. With characteristic generosity, Osler donated his honorarium to have these memorabilia properly bound and preserved.[33] Osler admired Harvey not only as a great physician and scientist but also as a great man who showed courage and persistence in the face of adversity.

While Osler admired Linacre for his scholarship and Harvey for his science, he more nearly resembled Thomas Sydenham, the "English Hippocrates," who although neither a great writer nor a great scientist, became famous as a generalist physician. Like Hippocrates, Sydenham contended that medicine should be based on observation and reasoning rather than philosophy and speculation. As Osler put it,

> Sydenham broke with authority and went to nature. It is extraordinary how he could have been so emancipated from dogmas and theories of all sorts. He laid down the fundamental proposition, and acted upon it, that "all disease could be described as natural history." [34]

Sydenham also taught that "nature alone often terminates diseases, and works a cure with a few simple medicines, and often enough with no medicines at all." [35] Osler hailed Sydenham as "a prince among practical physicians." [36] He also admired Sydenham's skepticism, saying that "Sydenham was called 'a man of many doubts' and therein lay the secret of his great strength." [37] Osler consciously became a meticulous observer of disease and a skeptic regarding most therapies of his day. Thus Osler admired "the men . . . who found for us the light and liberty of Greek thought—Linacre, Harvey, and Sydenham, those ancient founts of inspiration and models for all time in Literature, Science and Practice." [38]

Osler had many other heroes. For example, he admired John Locke, a physician who became a great philosopher. Locke's theories underlie much of what we take for granted in Western thought, including the notion, expressed in *The Declaration of Independence*, that all men are created equal. Osler noted:

> For each one of us there is still a "touch divine" in the life and writings of John Locke. A singularly attractive personality, with a sweet reasonableness of temper and a charming freedom from flaws and defects of character, he is an author whom we like at the first acquaintance, and soon love as a friend. Perhaps the greatest, certainly . . . the most characteristic English philosopher, we may claim Dr. Locke as a bright ornament of our profession.[39]

Osler admired the pioneering physicians of North America and often remembered them in his addresses to local medical societies. Speaking in Rhode Island, for example, he extolled the virtues of "Elisha Bartlett, teacher, philosopher, author . . . whom you may claim as the most distinguished physician of this State." [40] He called Boston's Oliver Wendell Holmes "the most successful combination the world has ever seen, of physician and man of letters." [41] He praised Philadelphia's William Pepper for

> the spirit in which [he] utilized his time in the service of his fellow men, and the chief lesson of his life to us who survive:
>
>> Contend, my soul, for moments and for hours;
>> Each is with service pregnant, each reclaimed
>> Is as a Kingdom conquered, where to reign.[42]

These examples illustrate Osler's ingrained habit of seeking out the finer attributes of others in order to become a better person himself.

At age 48, Osler made a clear statement about the importance of reference groups:

> Medicine is seen at its best in men whose faculties have had the highest and most harmonious culture. The Lathams, the Watsons, the Pagets, the Jenners, and the Gairdners have influenced the profession less by their special work than by exemplifying those graces of life and refinements of heart which make up character. And the men of this stamp in Greater Britain have left the most enduring mark,— Beaumont, Bovell and Hodder in Toronto; Holmes, Campbell and

Howard in this city [Montreal]; the Warrens, the Jacksons, the Bigelows, the Bowditches and the Shattucks in Boston; Bard, Hosack, Francis, Clark and Flint in New York; Morgan, Shippen, Redman, Rush, Coxe, the elder Wood, the elder Pepper, and the elder Mitchell of Philadelphia—Brahmins all, in the language of the greatest Brahmin among them, Oliver Wendell Holmes,—these and men like unto them have been the leaven which has raised our profession above the dead level of a business. [43]

Osler anchored his stand for professionalism in the examples of those he considered to have been great humanistic physicians. He recognized that the real importance of heroes is to find qualities that we, too, can absorb and that serve the interests of society as well as self.

TAKE ON PUPILS

Osler progressed through what are now seen as four stages of the mentor–protégé relationship. He began as an *apprentice* under such men as Johnson, Bovell, and Howard. He then became an *individual* contributor whose competence and originality showed in Montreal, Philadelphia, and Baltimore. As he rose rapidly in medicine's ranks, he became an increasingly effective *mentor,* especially during his Baltimore period. Finally, he matured into an *organization* influencer, one whose influence pervaded his institution and even his entire field.[44] Osler recognized that taking on pupils multiplies one's personal influence. Although he cultivated the older men of his time and revered the great figures of the past, he sought lasting impact through his pupils. His finest addresses, such as the essays that make up the *Aequanimitas* collection, were directed largely toward the young. Having been mentored by others, he became a mentor in turn.

From his first faculty appointment at age 25, Osler showed interest in his younger colleagues. Asked to give an introductory lecture to medical students, he told them:

You come now into the society not of mere professors, who will lecture at you from a distance, but of men who are anxious for your welfare, who will sympathize with your difficulties and also bear with your weakness. . . . Look upon us as elder brothers to whom you can come confidently and fearlessly for advice in any trouble or difficulty.[45]

But he matured fully into the role of mentor only in his fifth decade—an age that we now associate with the ability to assume this role.[46] His 1892 marriage to Grace Revere Gross, the widow of a Philadelphia surgeon, helped a great deal (see Chapter 8). She not only assumed the spousal role of career strategist, but also enabled him to create a home atmosphere similar to what he had known with Bovell in Toronto and Howard in Montreal. The couple's house at One West Franklin Street became a haven for medical students. Osler gave especially promising young men latchkeys so that they might come and go as they pleased in his large and growing personal library. The "latch-keyers," as they came to be known, seldom enjoyed the intense one-on-one relationship that Osler had known with Johnson, Bovell, and Howard, possibly because Osler was by then famous and deemed it best not to play favorites. Osler was a good judge of people and showed "remarkable skill or good luck" in choosing those whom he especially wanted to inspire.[47] However, all of the latch-keyers knew they were special. Those who went to Europe to study were even given gold wedding bands to wear "as a form of protection against any designing and matrimonially minded Gretel they might encounter while sojourning on the Continent." [48]

Osler gave students access to his time as well as to his library. By age 47, he had begun a custom of spending Saturday evenings in their company. Two senior students would be invited to One West Franklin Street at seven o'clock, and the others would be invited to come an hour later. Osler asked them about their patients and about what they had learned from their reading. He then served beer with biscuits and cheese and entertained them by reading from a favorite author from medicine or literature. Harvey Cushing concluded that "in these surroundings he was at his best." [49] Osler took pleasure in showing the students his old medical books. If the students were delighted by the books, they were even more gratified by their professor's warmth and enthusiasm.

Why did Osler choose to spend Saturday evenings with medical students? Would it not have served him better to enjoy cultural events or Baltimore society? Perhaps he opted for the students

because of his principles and priorities. Perhaps he felt that being
with them was more fun:

> Except it be a lover, no one is more interesting as an object of study
> than a student. Shakespeare might have made him a fourth in his
> immortal group. The lunatic with his fixed idea, the poet with his fine
> frenzy, the lover with his frantic idolatry, and the student aflame with
> the desire for knowledge are of "imagination all compact." . . .
> Like the Snark, he defies definition, but there are three unmistakable
> signs by which you may recognize the genuine article from a Boo-
> jum—an absorbing desire to know the truth, an unswerving stead-
> fastness in its pursuit, and an open, honest heart, free from suspi-
> cion, guile, and jealousy.[50]

Or perhaps it was because of his own need for stimulation:

> Men above forty are rarely pioneers, rarely the creators in science
> or in literature. The work of the world has been done by men who
> had not reached *la crise de quarante ans* [the crisis of forty years;
> mid-life crisis]. And in our profession wipe out, with but few excep-
> tions, the contributions of men above this age and we remain
> essentially as we are. Once across this line we teachers and consult-
> ants are in constant need of post-graduate study as an antidote
> against premature senility. Daily contact with the bright young
> minds of our associates and assistants, the mental friction of medi-
> cal societies, and travel are important aids.[51]

Osler knew that good mentors showcase their protégés' skills and
accomplishments. He encouraged students to report their observations in the medical literature and become scholars in their own
right. He praised and even spotlighted their published work. Thus
when he came across a case report by young O. H. Perry Pepper,
son of his deceased Philadelphia colleague William Pepper, in an
obscure local journal, Osler not only sent a short congratulatory
note but also wrote a long annotation about Pepper's article for
Britain's most prestigious journal, the *Lancet*.[52] Unlike some of his
contemporaries, Osler believed firmly that students deserved due
credit for their findings. Thayer paraphrased him as having said:

> Let every student have full recognition for his work. Never hide the
> work of others under your own name. Should your assistant make
> an important observation, let him publish it. Through your students
> and your disciples will come your greatest honor.[53]

Like most if not all male professors of his day, Osler used the masculine pronouns "him" or "his" in describing medical students. However, he was not oblivious to women in the profession. Early in his career, Osler indicated that "my sympathies are entirely with them in the attempt to work out the problem as to how far they can succeed in such an arduous profession as that of medicine." [54] Later, the Johns Hopkins University School of Medicine opened with the stipulation that women be admitted on equal footing with men. Osler wrote:

> For years I have been waiting the advent of the modern Trotula [a woman or women associated with the medical school at Salerno in Italy during the Middle Ages], a woman in the profession with an intellect so commanding that she will rank with the Harveys, the Hunters, and Pasteurs; the Virchows, and the Listers. That she has not yet arisen is no reflection on the small band of women physicians who have joined our ranks in the last fifty years. Stars of the first magnitude are rare, but that such a one will arise among women physicians I have not the slightest doubt. And let us be thankful that when she comes she will not have to waste her precious energies in the worry of a struggle for recognition. [55]

More fundamentally, he believed that there was a great need for change in medical education and that one highly desirable change was that *all* teachers should assume the attitude of fellow students:

> The successful teacher is no longer on a height, pumping knowledge at high pressure into passive receptacles. The new methods have changed all this. He is no longer *Sir Oracle*, perhaps unconsciously by his very manner antagonizing minds to whose level he cannot possibly descend, but he is a senior student anxious to help his juniors. When a simple, earnest spirit animates a college, there is no appreciable interval between the teacher and the taught—both are in the same class, the one a little more advanced than the other. So animated, the student feels that he has joined a family whose honour, whose welfare is his own, and whose interests should be his first consideration. [56]

Osler kept up with many of his former students and formed close relationships with a few. One of these few was Charles N. B. Camac, a graduate of the University of Pennsylvania School of Medicine, who was a resident at Johns Hopkins between 1895 and 1897—Osler's prime. In 1905, after the Oslers had moved to

Oxford, Camac spent several weeks with them, during which he worked with Osler toward distilling the *Counsels and Ideals* from Osler's writings.[57] Camac thus honored Osler and, in doing so, extended his mentor's influence.

In a eulogy of Osler, it was said that he "achieved many honours and many dignities, but the proudest of all was his unwritten title, 'the Young Man's Friend.' " [58]

SHOW GRATITUDE

Osler made clear his gratitude to his teachers, colleagues, and students on various occasions. On May 2, 1905, at a farewell dinner in New York given "by the profession of the United States and Canada" as he prepared to leave for England, he attributed his happiness largely to his interpersonal relationships:

> Happiness comes to many of us and in many ways, but I can truly say that to few men has happiness come in so many forms as it has come to me. Why I know not, but this I do know, that I have not deserved more than others, and yet, a very rich abundance of it has been vouchsafed to me. . . . I have had exceptional happiness in the profession of my choice, and I owe all of this to you. I have sought success in life, and if, as some one has said, this consists in getting what you want and being satisfied with it, I have found what I wanted in the estimation, in the fellowship and friendship of the members of my profession.[59]

He also thanked his students, saying, "My relations with my students—so many of whom I see here—have been of a close and most friendly character. They have been the inspiration of my work, and I may say truly, the inspiration of my life." [60]

In a farewell address to the Maryland State Medical Society, Osler similarly credited his success to serving others:

> As an untried young man my appointment at McGill College came directly through friends in the faculty who had confidence in me as a student. In the ten years I lived in Montreal I saw little of any save physicians and students, among whom I was satisfied to work—and to play. In Philadelphia the hospitals and the societies absorbed the greater part of my time, and I lived the peaceful life of a student with students. An ever-widening circle of friends in the profession

brought me into closer contact with the public, but I have never departed from my ambition to be first of all a servant of my brethren, willing and anxious to do anything in my power to help them.[61]

And in July 1919, at an international celebration of his seventieth birthday, he said:

> To have had the benediction of friendship follow me like a shadow, to have always had the sense of comradeship in work without the petty pinpricks of jealousies and controversies, to be able to rehearse in the sessions of sweet, silent thought the experiences of long years without a single bitter memory fill the heart with gratitude. That three transplantations have been borne successfully I owe to the brotherly care with which you have tended me. Loving our profession and believing ardently in its future I have been content to live in it and for it. A moving ambition to become a good teacher and a sound clinician was fostered by opportunities of exceptional character and any success I may have attained must be attributed in large part to the unceasing kindness of colleagues and to a long series of devoted pupils whose success in life is my special pride.[62]

Osler thus tacitly acknowledged that however great our personal productivity might be, happiness comes mainly from our bonds with other humans. He omitted the obvious: his fellowships and friendships were richly earned.

Although Osler freely expressed his gratitude, he acknowledged that ingratitude is all too often the norm. He noted, "It is a common experience that men do not always appreciate their blessings and advantages. Those who are the best off are the least sensible of it." [63] He may have consciously guarded against this tendency for, as it was observed, "No one who showed him a kindness was ever forgotten." [64] He often arranged complimentary dinners, suggested gifts or portraits, or simply included others in his activities. He did not require that the beneficiaries of his largesse should be able to reciprocate his favors. For example, he sponsored a gift for a male nurse who had lived in Philadelphia's "Old Blockley" hospital for 30 years. Cushing observed that among Osler's "great charms was the kindly interest he took in obscure workers in any field of medicine." [65] Moreover, he "had an unerring flair which enabled him to foresee before others when words of encouragement or appreciation were needed, and when appropriate." [66]

Osler thus made a habit of affirming others and boosting their self-esteem. The extent to which he was honored and affirmed in turn substantiates the truism that the best way to impress others is to show that we are impressed by them. The testimonials that he received when he left North America were also testimonials to the principles of good interpersonal relationships. Osler built his career on balancing work with personal relationships and, like most people, found that sustained happiness nearly always comes from helping others, not ourselves.

UNDERSTAND THE CHEMISTRY

Today's literature on mentoring acknowledges many types of mentors and mentor-protégé relationships. Formally defined as "a highly complex people-related skill, involving comprehensive concern for life-adjustment behavior," mentoring has been evaluated, classified, and subclassified from many points of view.[67] Some types of mentors, such as the "unknown sponsor" relationship, carry few if any risks to either party. However, the classic mentor-protégé relationship whereby the mentor serves as teacher, sponsor, adviser, and role model—sometimes called the godfather relationship—carries risks inherent in evolution that resemble those of romantic love. Mutual admiration gives way to shared vulnerability, setting the stage for disappointment. The best outcome is that the protégé becomes the mentor's peer. Psychologist Daniel Levinson concluded from his study of men that mentors are usually transitional figures in our lives and that the endings are typically painful for one or both parties.[68] Osler's relationships were not immune to these risks.

Osler's remarkable ability to form mentoring relationships reflected in part his innate ability to understand people, which in turn reflected the advantage of having been the youngest son in a large, close-knit family. Edith Reid observed that the "psychological instinct of Dr. Osler was entirely intuitive, unsought; and in contrast to his pathological work, not laboriously developed." [69] His keen sense of humor no doubt helped. Osler was fun to be around, and perhaps it was his sense of humor that enabled him to break through Palmer Howard's stern demeanor. Osler's loyalty to his mentors was shown by his never changing the dedication page to *The Principles and Practice of Medicine* despite the book's extensive revisions during his lifetime. But what were the final outcomes of his relationships with the three men to whom he dedicated the book: Johnson, Bovell, and Howard? Were the end results joy or regret?

Father Johnson seems to have harbored at least a measure of bitterness. Perhaps he was disappointed that Osler chose medicine over the ministry. When Johnson's own son became a medical student at McGill after Osler had taken a teaching position there, Johnson congratulated him on maintaining a distance from his former pupil:

> I am not surprised at your not taking up with Professor Osler. He is an Osler, and there is that in him, unless I am mistaken, which you must never admire. He wanted me to let you board with him, but I never encouraged the idea. . . . I would like to write you a good deal on the Osler character. . . . There does not appear to be any talent about them, or any high principle of action. Simply great application, and, probably the motive is money making.[70]

So far as is known, Osler never criticized Johnson. Yet one is left to wonder whether Osler perceived a special quality in the relationship that, in the end, was not there.

Osler never saw James Bovell again after the latter's return to the West Indies. Osler regarded Bovell as something of an alter ego, and for the rest of his life, when his mind drifted as it was likely to do during a dull committee meeting, he was apt to doodle "James Bovell" or "James Bovell, M.D., M.R.C.P." He appreciated Bovell especially for stimulating his interest in books:

> Books and the Man! The best the human mind has afforded was on his [Bovell's] shelves, and in him all that one could desire in a teacher, a clear head and a loving heart. Infected with the Aesculapian spirit, he made me realize the truth of those memorable words in the Hippocratic oath, "I will honour as my father the man who teaches me the Art." [71]

However, he did not hesitate to criticize Bovell's diffuseness:

> Only men of a certain metal rise superior to their surroundings, and while Dr. Bovell had that all-important combination of boundless ambition with energy and industry, he had that fatal fault of diffuse-

ness, in which even genius is strangled. With a quadrilateral mind, which he kept spinning like a teetotum, one side was never kept uppermost for long at a time. Caught in a storm which shook the scientific world with the publication of the *Origin of Species*, instead of sailing before the wind, even were it with bare poles, he put about and sought a harbour of refuge in writing a work on Natural Theology, which you will find on the shelves of second-hand book shops in a company made respectable at least by the presence of Paley.[72]

Palmer Howard continued to be a father figure for Osler, but the emotional bonds between the two were never so close as the bonds between Osler and Bovell had been. At age 23, Osler had the courage to stand up to Howard after the latter had arranged for him to be offered the chair in botany at McGill. Osler recognized that the appointment would not help him with his career path, and he therefore wrote Howard:

I am afraid you will not be pleased at it, but I really can not do otherwise. If I knew anything of Botany at present; if I had nothing else left to do for three or four years it might be thought of; but as matters stand now I would only make a fool of myself in accepting such a position. I would feel far too keenly the anomalous situation of holding a chair in Botany & knowing absolutely nothing of the Flora of my native land.[73]

Perhaps it was because of these experiences that Osler formed few intense personal mentor relationships with members of the younger generation. His approach to mentoring was largely utilitarian in that he sought to influence many (perhaps all) of the promising younger people who surrounded him rather than a chosen few. An exception was Harvey Cushing, a surgical resident whom Osler took under his wing possibly because he saw in Cushing a mirror image of himself. Cushing's relationship to Osler progressed from protégé to friend to admiring biographer.[74] However, Osler, too, expressed disappointment about the outcomes of many of his former protégés:

From one cause or another, perhaps because when not absorbed in the present, my thoughts are chiefly in the past, I have cherished the memory of many young men whom I have loved and lost. *Io victis*: let us sometimes sing of the vanquished. Let us sometimes think of those who have fallen in the battle of life, who have striven and failed, who have failed even without the strife. How many have I lost from the student band by mental death, and from so many causes—some stillborn from college, others dead within the first year of infantile marasmus, while mental rickets, teething, tabes, and fits have carried off many of the most promising minds!

Even worse than mental death was moral death:

> To the teacher-nurse it is a sore disappointment to find at the end of ten years so few minds within the full stature, of which the early days gave promise. Still, so widespread is mental death that we scarcely comment upon it in our friends. The real tragedy is the moral death which, in different forms, overtakes as many good fellows who fall away from the pure, honourable, and righteous service of Minerva into the idolatry of Bacchus, of Venus, and of Circe.

Such moral death was even worse than the physical deaths of former students, although these, too, deeply affected him:

> Less painful to dwell upon, though associated with a more poignant grief, is the fate of those whom physical death has snatched away in the bud or blossom of the student life. These are among the tender memories of the teacher's life, of which he does not often care to speak, feeling with Longfellow that the surest pledge of their remembrance is "the silent homage of thoughts unspoken." [75]

Despite such disappointments, Osler found with time that keeping up with former protégés brought him some of his greatest satisfactions. Cushing noted that "Osler's deep interest in the welfare of all his associates and assistants, past and present" was a salient aspect of the short notes and letters that Osler habitually dashed off to such persons. Hundreds of such notes and letters still exist. Usually undated and consisting of but a few sentences, they show his ongoing "concern for their work and prospects, after they had gone out from under his wing." [76] Osler's relationships with both mentors and protégés illustrate the truisms that friendships require work, that affirmation ranks high among our basic human needs, and that—ultimately—happiness hinges not on achievement but rather on the range and depth of our relationships with others.

4

BE

POSITIVE

"Prince of Friends and Benefactors"

Contemporaries summed up William Osler's approach to life with such adjectives as alert, boyish, buoyant, cheerful, interested, and vivacious, to name a few. Today, we would say "upbeat." Several of the people who knew him best, however, felt that he was to some extent a chronic depressive. One wrote, "Osler had a sad face, and I have always suspected that there was a good deal of sadness underneath this extremely jovial exterior." [1] Osler's fascination with *The Anatomy of Melancholy*, a colorful treatise published in 1621 by Robert Burton, an English clergyman who tried to write his way out of depression, supports this suggestion. But Osler hid any possible depressive tendencies remarkably well. His trademark positive attitude featured optimism, generosity, diligence, decisiveness, tolerance, and—perhaps most important of all—selective use of the more mature psychological defense mechanisms.

BE AN OPTIMIST

From the biblical writers and the Stoic philosophers of antiquity to such twentieth-century motivational speakers as Earl Nightingale and Norman Vincent Peale runs this truism: We become what we think about. Osler's shadow presence, Sir Thomas Browne, expressed the essence of positive thinking: "Let the Characters of good things stand indelibly in thy Mind, and thy Thoughts be active on them." [2] Emerson was similarly emphatic: "As a man thinketh, so is he, and as a man chooseth, so is he and so is nature." [3] Speaking to medical students, Osler echoed Abraham Lincoln's reflection that most people are about as happy as they make up their minds to be:

> To each one of you the practice of medicine will be very much as you make it—to one a worry, a care, a perpetual annoyance; to another, a daily joy and a life of as much happiness and usefulness as can well fall to the lot of man.[4]

By most accounts, Osler was positive thinking personified. Although his sunny disposition was to a large extent constitutional, dating to early childhood, he cultivated several traits that anyone can adopt. First, he sought to eliminate negative phenomena from his speech, his writing, and presumably, his thoughts. He understood that the more we talk about unpleasantness—accidents, crime, deaths, disasters, and so forth—the more we are likely to become negative people ourselves. He warned against complaining:

> *You may learn to consume your own smoke.* The atmosphere is darkened by the murmurings and whimperings of men and women over the nonessentials, the trifles that are inevitably incident to the hurly burly of the day's routine. Things cannot always go your way. Learn to accept in silence the minor aggravations, cultivate the gift of taciturnity and consume your own smoke with an extra draught of hard work, so that those about you may not be annoyed with the dust and soot of your complaints.[5]

Looking away from negative phenomena was a facet of his famous equanimity (see Chapter 6):

> It has been said that "in patience ye shall win your souls," and what is this patience but an equanimity which enables you to rise superior to the trials of life? Sowing as you shall do beside all waters, I can but wish that you may repeat the promised blessing of quietness and assurance forever, until
>
> Within this life,
> Though lifted o'er its strife,
>
> you may, in the growing winters, glean a little of that wisdom which is pure, peaceable, gentle, full of mercy and good fruits, without partiality and without hypocrisy.[6]

In a draft of one of his essays, he told of the death of his younger sister, Emma—the last child born to Featherstone Lake and Ellen Pickton Osler. Although this death may have haunted him throughout life, he edited the passage out of the final version. Why? He wished to spare himself and others from the harmful effects of negative emotions.

Second, he celebrated life by dwelling on the positive. This was not easy, as the medical wards of his day were lined with patients suffering from tuberculosis, typhoid fever, and pneumonia for which there were no effective therapies. Osler encouraged physicians and nurses with the message that

> suffering and disease are ever before us, but life is very pleasant; and the motto of the world, when well, is "forward with the dance." Fondly imagining that we are in a happy valley, we deal with ourselves as the King did with the Gautama, and hide away everything that suggests our fate. Perhaps we are wise. Who knows? Mercifully, the tragedy of life, though seen, is not realized. It is so close that we lose all sense of its proportions.[7]

It was in this context that the great Rockefeller Institute scientist René Dubos mentioned Osler prominently in his essay "The Despairing Optimist." [8] From the wards filled with terrible infections, Osler looked away toward the triumphs of public health:

> These are glorious days for the race. Nothing has been seen like it on this old earth since the destroying angel stayed his hand on the

threshing-floor of Araunah the Jebusite. For seven years, Cuba, once a pest-house of the tropics, has been free from scourge [yellow fever] which has left an indelible mark in the history of the Englishman, Spaniard, and American in the New World.[9]

As noted earlier, this strain of optimism reflected in part Osler's living during the Progressive Era, in which human progress was seen as more nearly linear than we see it today (see Chapter 2). However, he believed that in two areas—physical well-being and, to a lesser extent, individual rights—people had seldom if ever been better off:

> Of practical progress . . . there can be no doubt; no one can dispute the enormous increase in the comfort of each individual life. Collectively the human race, or portions of it at any rate, may in the past have enjoyed periods of greater repose, and longer intervals of freedom from strife and anxiety; but the day has never been when the unit has been of such value, when the man, and the man alone, has been so much the measure, when the individual as a living organism has seemed so sacred, when the obligations to regard his rights have seemed so imperative. But even these changes are as nothing in comparison with the remarkable increase in his physical well-being. The bitter cry of Isaiah that with the multiplication of the nations their joys have not been increased, still echoes in our ears. The sorrows and troubles of men, it is true, may not have been materially diminished, but bodily pain and suffering, though not abolished, have been assuaged as never before.[10]

A third aspect of Osler's optimism was that he sought to take charge of his life and to strive constantly toward definite goals, to control events rather than be controlled by them. People who knew him at each stage of life found him the model of a happy, optimistic person. His forward-looking image began with his dress, which was neither extravagant nor vain but always neat and appropriate. He took pride in his large collection of colorful cravats and neckties, kept a flower in his buttonhole, and carried his walking stick and yellow kid gloves with a flare. His pace was quick and buoyant. His "fate was always to move a step higher, and never to look back with regret on a step once taken." [11] He epitomized self-reliance as taught by Emerson, who said among other things: "Shallow men believe in luck. . . . Strong men believe in cause and effect." [12]

Fourth, Osler projected the positive image of a person primarily concerned about others, living out the philosophy that *"we are here not to get all we can out of life for ourselves, but to try to make the lives of others happier."* [13] He recognized that a sure formula for happiness is to lose oneself in a life of service to others. This was indeed the advice of the great twentieth-century psychiatrist, Karl Menninger, who suggested that a good remedy for depression is to go to the other side of the railroad tracks and start helping the less fortunate. Osler told his students that the hardest lesson of all is that *"the law of the higher life is only fulfilled by love, i.e. charity."* He felt strongly that one should be charitable toward other physicians:

> Many a physician whose daily work is a daily round of beneficence will say hard things and think hard thoughts of a colleague. No sin will so easily beset you as uncharitableness towards your brother practitioner. So strong is the personal element in the practice of medicine, and so many are the wagging tongues in every parish that evil-speaking, lying, and slandering find a shining mark in the lapses and mistakes which are inevitable in our work. There is no reason for discord and disagreement, and the only way to avoid trouble is to have two plain rules. From the day you begin practice never under any circumstances listen to a tale told to the detriment of a brother practitioner. And when any dispute or trouble does arise, go frankly, ere sunset, and talk the matter over, in which way you may gain a brother and a friend.[14]

On another occasion, he told students to "never listen to a patient who begins with a story about the carelessness and inefficiency of Dr. Blank." [15] He summed up this attitude of charity in three words: "Respect your colleagues." [16]

It was no coincidence that Osler's bedside reading list for medical students included two of the great Stoic philosophers, Marcus Aurelius and Epictetus. The essence of their advice was that we cannot always control events but can we control our attitudes. Osler paraphrased the great Stoics when he said, "Even with disaster ahead and ruin imminent, it is better to face them with a smile, and with the head erect, than to crouch at their approach." [17] The Latin root of "optimism" means "best." Osler taught and practiced positive thinking, having made a conscious decision that optimism, if adequately grounded in reality, is invariably the better strategy than its alternative.

BE GENEROUS

Most positive people give generously, and Osler was no exception. Even as a boy, he "was quick to give the last penny of his scant pocket-money to another who might be hard up." [18] Yet he was mindful that good intentions need monitoring. Sir Thomas Browne had written, "I must confess I am charitable only in my liberal intentions, and bountiful well-wishes." [19] Still, Osler admired Browne as a "prudent, prosperous man, generous to his children and to his friends," who "subscribed liberally to his old school in Winchester, to the rebuilding of the Library of Trinity College, Cambridge, and to the repairs at Christ Church, Oxford." [20] Many people testified that Osler was similarly generous throughout his life.

At age 25, he found himself teaching physiology and histology to medical students at McGill. There were not enough micro-scopes to go around. Osler had little money to spare but was receiving a stipend of five hundred dollars for taking charge of the smallpox ward. He used the entire sum to buy microscopes for the students. As he later explained it:

> The students paid fees directly to the instructors, who provided equipment and material and lived on the balance. I did more of the former and less of the latter. The supply of microscopes was meagre, and after remedying this defect there was little left in my pockets.[21]

His cousin Marian Osborne told a remarkable story of Osler's McGill days in which the young professor literally gave his coat to a stranger:

> We were dancing along St. Catherine Street hand in hand, when an old and very seedy-looking man accosted us and asked for money. Uncle Bill looked at him with his penetrating brown eyes and said with a laugh—"You old rascal, why should I give you money to drink yourself to death?" "Well Sir, it lightens the road going." "There is only one thing of value about you and that is your hobnailed liver." "I'll give it to you, Sir. I'll give it to you." Dr. Osler laughed and putting his hand in his pocket drew out some silver which he gave to the old man saying: "Now, Jehosaphat, promise me you will get some soup before you start in on the gin." The old fellow eagerly agreed and went away with infirmity in his step. The doctor looked after him with a thoughtful expression. "Pretty cold for that poor

fellow," he murmured and then I found we were running after the beggar. "Here, take this. I have a father of my own," said the doctor pulling off his overcoat and putting it on the astonished old man. "You may drink yourself to death and undoubtedly will, but I cannot let you freeze to death." "Tell me your name, Sir." "William Osler, and don't forget to leave me that liver." With a wave of his hand we continued on our dancing way. Virtue was rewarded two weeks later. The old man, before he died in the hospital, made his last will and testament, leaving his "hobnailed liver and his overcoat to his good friend William Osler!" [22]

There were numerous less dramatic examples of Osler's giving. He was especially generous to children, often bringing them small favors and showing "an amusing proclivity for giving children nicknames," one of his trademarks.[23] In his later life, few things brought him more pleasure than giving a valuable rare book to a library or fellow collector.[24] When he went to Europe, he sometimes bought books with such "reckless generosity" that he had a hard time paying the fare for his return to England.[25]

Osler admired generosity in others. Of his Johns Hopkins colleague Howard A. Kelly, he said: "He was exceedingly liberal and gave with great freedom both to the Hospital, to his assistants, and to general charities." Of William H. Welch, he likewise wrote: "A more unselfish man never lived—his time, his brain, his books, his purse were at the command of all." [26] Osler multiplied his personal generosity by being an effective fundraiser, especially for libraries. In 1897, for example, he encouraged Maryland physicians to donate for this purpose:

May I say a word on the art of giving? The essence is contained in the well-known sentence, "let every man do according as he is disposed in his heart, not grudgingly or of necessity." Subscriptions to a cause which is for the benefit of the entire profession should truly be given as a man is disposed in his heart, not in his pocket, and assuredly not of necessity, but as a duty, even as a privilege, and as a pleasure. Some of us, the younger men, cannot give. The days of travail and distress are not yet over, and to give would be wrong. It is sufficient for such to have the wish to give; the elder brothers will bear your share; only be sure to foster those generous impulses, which are apt to be intense in direct proportion to the emptiness of the purse.[27]

A Baltimore colleague showed his appreciation for Osler's generosity:

> I think to have a big generous heart and then to have the means of making it happy through generous acts and deeds is the nearest approach to Heaven we can get in this life. I never saw a man who enjoyed giving as much as you do, and I presume this is one reason why you are always happy. If I should outlive you I will make the old Faculty erect a monument to your memory if I have to give all the money myself. I rejoice with you in the good work you are doing.[28]

A British colleague of the newly arrived Canadian described how Osler, at 56, had taken Oxford by storm with his energy, generosity, and positive thinking:

> Though Oxford is proverbially hospitable and generous, she does not easily capitulate to strangers, especially if their claim to distinction rests upon scientific rather than on literary grounds, but Osler left Oxford no choice, and from the first the surrender of the university was absolute and immediate. Of course his great reputation as a physician and medical writer had preceded him, but we immediately discovered that finished competence in his own art and science was but a small part of the man, that the new Regius Professor was the least professional of doctors and the least academic of professors, that he was amazingly devoid of vanity and pedantic inhibitions, that his spirit was free, alert, vivacious, and that there was apparently no end to the span of his interests or to the vivid life-giving energy which he was prepared to throw into any task which fell to him to discharge. Old and young alike acknowledged his mastery and never left his presence without feeling the magnetism of the man and that insatiable, but unobtrusive appetite for helpfulness which made him the prince of friends and benefactors.[29]

Predictably, the example of Osler's generosity prompted many of his contemporaries to become deeply involved in public-spirited activities.[30]

WORK

Osler's capacity for work was legendary among his contemporaries; as Cushing put it, "His industry was proverbial." Osler's dedication and persistence soon became apparent after he took a faculty position at McGill. Concentrating on autopsy pathology, he made careful dissections, completed the reports in his own handwriting, assembled a huge compendium of observations, and built a medical museum.[31] This work was the basis for his mastery of medicine, which was in turn the basis for his later fame and influence. But Osler's work at Montreal was hardly confined to autopsies. He studied and taught biology and physiology as well as pathology, supported a club for medical students, brought new life to a sleepy medical society, and wrote scores of articles for the medical literature. He showed courage by taking charge of the smallpox wards, charity in his dealings with his fellow physicians in and out of his school, generosity to his students, and fidelity to his sundry tasks to the extent that "his many uncommon qualities had earned him popularity unsought and of a most unusual degree." [32] In the best sense of the term, he hustled.

Like most highly successful people, Osler followed the rule that one should always do more than one is paid or expected to do. He urged students to bring to their work both passion and a high energy level:

> To an absorbing passion, a whole-souled devotion, must be joined an enduring energy, if the student is to become a devotee of the grey-eyed goddess to whose law his services are bound.[33]

In 1903 he gave a lecture to students at the University of Toronto entitled "The Master-Word of Medicine." What word would it be? As the students listened expectantly, Osler heightened the tension:

> It seems a bounden duty on such an occasion to be honest and frank, so I propose to tell you the secret of life as I have seen the game played and as I have tried to play it myself. You remember in one of the Jungle Stories that when Mowgli wished to be avenged on the villagers he could only get the help of Hathi and his sons by sending them the master-word. This I propose to give you in the hope, yes, in the full assurance, that some of you at least will lay hold upon it to your profit. Though a little one, the master-word looms large in meaning. It is the open sesame to every portal, the great equalizer in the world, the true philosopher's stone, which transmutes all the base metal of humanity into gold. The stupid among you it will make bright, the bright man brilliant, and the brilliant student steady. With the magic word in your heart all things

are possible, and without it all study is vanity and vexation. The miracles of life are with it; the blind see by touch, the deaf hear with eyes, the dumb speak with fingers. To the youth it brings hope, to the middle-aged confidence, to the aged repose. True balm of hurt minds, in its presence the heart of the sorrowful is lightened and consoled. It is directly responsible for all advances in medicine during the past twenty-five centuries.

After this eloquent preamble, Osler served up the secret of life:

And the master-word is *Work*, a little one, as I have said, but fraught with momentous sequences if you can but write it on the tablets of your hearts, and bind it upon your foreheads. But there is a serious difficulty in getting you to understand the paramount importance of the work-habit as part of your organization. You are not far from the Tom Sawyer stage with its philosophy "that work consists of whatever a body is obliged to do, and that play consists of whatever a body is not obliged to do." [34]

When he called work (rather than sleep, as Shakespeare had) the "true balm of hurt minds," Osler hit upon the truism that it is hard to be busy and depressed at the same time. In another classic essay, "A Way of Life," he similarly observed:

Steady work . . . gives a man a sane outlook on the world. No corrective [is] so valuable to the weariness, the fever, and the fret that are so apt to wring the heart of the young. This is the talisman, as George Herbert says,

> The famous stone
> That turneth all to gold,

and with which, to the eternally recurring question, What is Life? you answer, I do not think—I act it; the only philosophy that brings you in contact with its real values and enables you to grasp its hidden meaning. Over the Slough of Despond, past Doubting Castle and Giant Despair, with this talisman you may reach the Delectable Mountains, and those Shepherds of the Mind—Knowledge, Experience, Watchful, and Sincere.[35]

Since Osler's time, the word "workaholic" has been coined to describe those who seem unable to enjoy other aspects of life on account of their obsessions with their jobs. Osler enjoyed companionship and laughter at least as much as most people. But as a young man, he made a conscious decision to block out various "pursuits and pleasures" so that he could excel as a physician:

> In the first place, acquire early the *Art of Detachment*, by which I mean the faculty of isolating yourselves from the pursuits and pleasures incident to youth. By nature man is the incarnation of idleness, which quality alone, amid the ruined remnants of Edenic characters, remains in all its primitive intensity. Occasionally we do find an individual who takes to toil as others to pleasure, but the majority of us have to wrestle hard with the original Adam, and find it no easy matter to scorn delights and live laborious days.[36]

Although he usually made it look easy, he no doubt wrestled hard with how to balance work and play. His basic method was to set aside blocks of protected time for focused work while making sure that he also spent time with the people around him. In Philadelphia, he gained the reputation of being "hard to find," but "when found and an appointment made he was scrupulously punctual."[37] This was no accident for he held that "punctuality is the prime essential of a physician—if invariably on time he will succeed even in the face of professional mediocrity."[38] He also recognized the enormous value of persistence and determination. Thus in Osler's obituary of Richard Lea MacDonnell, he observed that to MacDonnell's natural gifts "were added those mental gifts which alone assure success—industry and perseverance."[39]

Indeed, in Osler's view there could be little or no excuse for not working hard toward long-term goals. Osler was extremely admiring of those whose careers had bloomed in seemingly barren soil:

> Some of the most brilliant work has been done by men in extremely limited spheres of action, and during the past hundred years it is surprising how many of the notable achievements have been made by physicians dwelling far from educational centers—Jenner worked out his discovery in a village; McDowell, Long, and Sims were country doctors; Koch was a district physician.[40]

He admired people who, like him, defined themselves in part by their productivity. But he kept perspective by cultivating an inner calm based to a large extent on the classical literature. Biographer Edith Reid pointed out that as "you consider his life you get the impression of far too many functions, too much activity; in reading his essays you are in another realm, one of peace and beauty and assurance—the assurance of the preacher with the tolerance of the scholar." [41] Osler's secrets, then, were clear goals, hard work, and—to a greater extent than people realized—frequent reflection on his priorities.

BE DECISIVE

Osler's positive attitude carried over to an ability to make decisions quickly and confidently. This might explain, in part, his tendency not to worry, because worry usually reflects sustained fear caused by indecision. One contemporary gave this account of Osler:

> How well his friends remember the alert carriage and elastic tread, the soft, grave, playful manner, the ready quip, the fine deep-set eyes so dark, subtle and tender, the lofty well-moulded brow, and the air of decision and command which marked his bearing. He never appeared to be busy or fussed, or to find a situation intractable. He did not, to all appearance, allow small things to worry him, but moved smoothly forward, enjoying all the blessings of life, always resolute to take human nature at its best and to seize every occasion for kindness which the day might offer. [42]

Osler's life seems to illustrate the adage that major decisions are often easy if one has paid close attention to the small ones all along. His most prolonged hesitation about a big decision seems to have been at age 19, when he wavered over whether to leave preparation for the ministry in order to study medicine—possibly because he feared his parents' disappointment. [43] He admired decisiveness in others. In his obituary of Samuel W. Gross, the Philadelphia surgeon whose widow he married, he wrote, "In manner he was energetic and quick. In thought and discussion he at once went to the gist of a matter, and impressed all as a man of force and decided character." [44] In his ability to make decisions, Osler may again have been influenced by Sir Thomas Browne, who was quite blunt about our command to "perform the sober Acts and serious purposes of Man":

> Our hard entrance into the World, our miserable going out of it, our sicknesses, disturbances, and sad Rencounters in it, do clamorously tell us we come not into the World to run a Race of Delight, but to

perform the sober Acts and serious purposes of Man; which to omit were foully to miscarry in the advantage of humanity, to play away an unutterable Life, and to have lived in vain.[45]

Osler sometimes made snap decisions about such matters as buying a house. Deciding when to move to another city took a while longer. His move from Montreal to Philadelphia affords a lesson in decision-making technique. He was in Leipzig, Germany, when he received the letter offering the prestigious job as Chair of Clinical Medicine at the University of Pennsylvania. At first he thought the letter was a practical joke that someone had played on him in return for the countless jokes he had played on others (perhaps someone had purloined a piece of University of Pennsylvania stationery, and the whole thing was a hoax). Why leave McGill, where he knew everyone and felt at home? Then he received a cable asking him to meet Dr. S. Weir Mitchell of Philadelphia, who happened to be in Europe, to discuss the details of the appointment. Osler later recorded:

> I sat up late into the night balancing the pros and cons of Montreal and Philadelphia. In the former I had many friends, I loved the work and the opportunity was great. In the latter the field appeared very attractive, but it meant leaving many dear friends. I finally gave it up as unsolvable and decided to leave it to chance. I flipped a four-mark silver piece into the air. "Heads I go to Philadelphia; tails I remain at Montreal." It fell "heads." I went to the telegraph-office and wrote the telegram to Dr. Mitchell offering to go to Philadelphia. I reached in my pockets to pay for the wire. They were empty. My only change had been the four-mark piece which I had left as it had fallen on my table. It seemed like an act of Providence directing me to remain in Montreal. I half decided to follow the cue. Finally I concluded that inasmuch as I had placed the decision to chance I ought to abide by the turn of the coin, and returned to my hotel for it and sent the telegram.[46]

Although this story may have been embellished over time, it nonetheless illustrates several points about decision-making. First, Osler recognized that the decision was important and should be carefully weighed. Second, he used Benjamin Franklin's method of listing reasons for and against the action. Third, he grasped that making no decision at all might be worse than a poor decision. If by procrastination he left the search committee hanging, he would have tarnished his credibility among influential American physicians and thus jeopardized future prospects. Finally, he made the leap even though the ultimate choice seemed fraught with arbitrariness. A new wrinkle to the coin-toss method is to ask what one would *really like* the result to be and then choose accordingly. In another version of the story, Osler suggested that the initial offer had been provisional:

> Dr. Mitchell cabled me to meet him in London, as he and his good wife were commissioned to "look me over," particularly with reference to personal conditions. Dr. Mitchell said there was only one way in which the breeding of a man suitable for such a position, in such a city as Philadelphia, could be tested:—give him cherry pie and see how he disposed of the stones. I had read of the trick before and disposed of them genteelly in my spoon—and got the Chair![47]

Osler's decision to leave Philadelphia for Baltimore came more easily. He knew that the new medical school being planned at Johns Hopkins gave him the chance to organize a medical clinic and teaching program to his own specifications, unfettered by the past. He knew that excellent faculty members had already been recruited and that the chair of medicine was still available. He knew that he might be asked, since his reputation was growing. Dr. John Shaw Billings, a man of few words, was sent to Philadelphia to offer Osler the position. Osler later recalled of the visit:

> Without sitting down, he asked me abruptly, "Will you take charge of the medical department of The Johns Hopkins Hospital?" Without a moment's hesitation I answered, "Yes." "See Welch about the details; we are to open very soon. I am very busy to-day; good morning," and he was off, having been in my room not more than a couple of minutes.[48]

Osler was hugely successful in Baltimore, but eventually the price of fame proved high. He was in huge demand as a consultant and began to experience what we now call burnout. Thus his last major career decision was another logical one. He had been negotiating with the Oxford search committee for the position of Regius Professor of Medicine there and was offered the job. He wrote of the offer to his wife, who telegraphed: "DO NOT PROCRASTINATE ACCEPT AT ONCE." The matter was settled.[49]

BE TOLERANT OF OTHERS

Osler usually kept any negative opinions of others to himself, a practice that enhanced his own image as a positive person. Others feel safe around such people, for they know that they will not be criticized behind their backs. Howard A. Kelly put it succinctly: "It was his settled policy never to speak ill of anyone, but always to discover the good." [50] One of Osler's aphorisms was to "keep a looking glass in your own heart, and the more carefully you scan your own frailties, the more tender you are for those of your fellow creatures." [51] Tradition held that the sideboard in the Oslers' dining room was inscribed with an invisible motto: "If you cannot say anything good about a man, say nothing." [52] Whenever a disparaging or disrespectful remark of someone was made in his presence, he would quickly steer the conversation in a new direction by commenting on an unrelated subject. It was assumed that he had "so disciplined the direction of his thoughts that to think evil of a man's action was the same as thinking evil of one's own." [53]

Osler might have absorbed this admirable trait, like others, from his shadow presence, Sir Thomas Browne, who had four pieces of advice about interpersonal relations. The first was to refrain from criticizing others:

> No man can justly censure or condemn another, because indeed no man truly knows another. This I perceive in myself, for I am in the dark to all the world, and my nearest friends behold me but in a cloud; those that know me but superficially, think less of me than I do of myself; those of my near acquaintance think more; God, who truly knows me, knows that I am nothing.[54]

Second, one should try to find good in others:

> When you look upon the Imperfections of others, allow one Eye for what is Laudable in them, and the balance they have from some excellence, which may render them considerable.[55]

Third, one should not allow differences of opinion to alienate us from others:

> I could never divide myself from any man upon the difference of an opinion, or be angry with his judgement for not agreeing with me in that, from which perhaps within a few days I should dissent myself.[56]

And finally, one should be charitable:

> Now for that other Virtue of Charity, without which Faith is a mere
> notion, and of no existence, I have endeavoured to nourish the
> merciful disposition and humane inclination I borrowed from my
> Parents, and regulate it to the written and prescribed Laws of Char-
> ity; and if I hold the true Anatomy of myself, I am delineated and
> naturally framed to such a piece of virtue: for I am of a constitution
> so general, that it consorts and sympathizes with all things.[57]

Such advice served Osler well. He made countless friends and few
if any enemies.

Although Osler's gift for getting along with people was no
doubt due in part to the "people sense" he absorbed from his
parents and many siblings, he sharpened his skills by following
Browne's advice that we should be slow to judge. He gave a good
ground rule:

> One of the first essentials in securing a good-natured equanimity is
> not to expect too much of the people amongst whom you dwell.
> "Knowledge comes, but wisdom lingers," and in matters medical the
> ordinary citizen of to-day has not one whit more sense than the old
> Romans. . . . Deal gently then with this deliciously credulous old
> human nature in which we work, and restrain your indignation.[58]

He not only treated people gently but also resisted the temptation
to be drawn into arguments. He was often heard to chuckle to
himself after encounters with difficult people, "Glad to see you
come, and glad to see you go." He suggested that we give others
the benefit of the doubt whenever possible, being careful not to
judge them by our own standards:

> Curious, odd compounds are these fellow-creatures, at whose
> mercy you will be; full of fads and eccentricities, of whims and
> fancies; but the more closely we study their little foibles of one sort
> and another in the inner life which we see, the more surely is the
> conviction borne in upon us of the likeness of their weaknesses to
> our own. The similarity would be intolerable, if a happy egotism did
> not often render us forgetful of it. Hence the need of an infinite
> patience and of an ever-tender charity toward these fellow-crea-
> tures; have they not to exercise the same toward us?[59]

And he held back the temptation to fight back when being criticized. One observer put it, "He did not feel the pinpricks. Little

things are only great to little men. Dr. Osler was too big to notice them." [60]

Osler worked hard to spread goodwill in the medical profession, which was somewhat notorious for its acrimonious divisions. As he knew only too well,

> The wrangling and unseemly disputes which have too often disgraced our profession arise, in a great majority of cases, on the one hand, from this morbid sensitiveness to the confession of error, and, on the other, from a lack of brotherly consideration, and a convenient forgetfulness of our own failings.[61]

With time, his ability to influence his colleagues to take the high road became almost legendary. As the medical historian Fielding H. Garrison noted:

> What made him, in a very real sense, the ideal physician, the essential humanist of modern medicine, was his wonderful genius for friendship toward all and sundry; and, consequent upon this trait, his large, cosmopolitan spirit, his power of composing disputes and differences, of making peace upon the high places, of bringing about "Unity, Peace and Concord" among his professional colleagues. "Wherever Osler went," says one of his best pupils, "the charm of his personality brought men together; for the good in all men he saw, and as friends of Osler, all men met in peace." [62]

Osler once wrote a friend: "I suppose a good hater has his joys but he must have a good many uneasy moments which a man of my temperament escapes." [63] He recognized that we should be slow to criticize: "Exceptional men cannot be judged by ordinary standards." And indeed, it is best not to judge at all: "One special advantage of the sceptical attitude of mind is that a man is never vexed to find that after all he has been in the wrong." [64] Osler's secret to interpersonal relationships was that he was something of a latitudinarian, a person who tolerates a wide range of viewpoints.

Among the princes of history's latitudinarians was the seventeenth-century philosopher John Locke. Osler's fascination with Locke owed in part to Locke's having been a physician and a great friend of Thomas Sydenham, "the English Hippocrates." Locke is best known for *An Essay Containing Human Understanding*. His doctrine that all people are created equal is echoed in *The Declaration of Independence*, which reflects Locke's impact on the

Founding Fathers of the United States. Locke also wrote *Epistle on Toleration*. Osler said of Locke:

> As the apostle of common sense he may be ranked with Socrates and a few others who have brought philosophy from the clouds to the working-day world. Of his special virtues and qualifications as the typical English philosopher nothing need be said, but were there time I would fain dwell upon his character as a philanthropist—in the truest sense of the word. The author of the *Epistle on Toleration* . . . the man who wrote the memorable words, "All men are naturally in a state of freedom, also of equality," must be ranked as one of the great benefactors of the race.[65]

Osler especially praised Locke's *Fundamental Constitutions of the Government of Carolina*: "The celebrated clause, 'No person whatsoever shall disturb, molest, or prosecute another for his speculative opinions in religion or his way of worship,' expresses the spirit of toleration for which Locke strove all through his life." [66] Osler concluded that "Locke seems to have found a rule of life which I commend to you: 'Live the best life you can, but live it so as not to give needless offence to others; do all you can to avoid the vices, follies, and weaknesses of your neighbours, but take no needless offence at their divergences from your ideal.' " [67] This was, in essence, Osler's own doctrine of tolerance for his fellow humans.

USE THE MATURE DEFENSES

Long-term observations by the psychiatrist George E. Vaillant and his colleagues suggest that success, however measured, depends critically on two factors: our relationships with other people and our choice of defense mechanisms (also called adaptive mechanisms).[68] In what came to be known as the Harvard Old Boy Study or the Grant Study, these investigators evaluated a large group of Harvard undergraduates between 1937 and 1944 and then followed them for more than 30 years. They concluded that our defenses against stresses and strains of life can be arranged into four groups:

1. *Psychotic mechanisms* (common in psychosis, dreams, and childhood)—denial of external reality, distortion, and delusional projection

2. *Immature mechanisms* (common in severe depression, personality disorders, and adolescence)—fantasy, projection, hypo-
   chondriasis, passive-aggressive behavior, and acting out
3. *Neurotic mechanisms* (common in everyone)—intellectualiza-
   tion, repression, reaction formation, and dissociation or neurotic denial
4. *Mature mechanisms* (common in healthy adults): sublimation,
   altruism, suppression, anticipation, and humor.

The men who habitually used the more mature defenses were by
far the most successful by every parameter studied: happiness,
income, rich friendships, harmonious marriage, and both mental
and physical health. Unfortunately, the investigators concluded,
the more mature defenses cannot be readily taught. However, they
can be absorbed from the people around us, and we can consciously seek to use sublimation, altruism, and humor.

William Osler was no stranger to stress and depression. He
spoke even of "the stress of routine class and laboratory duties." [69]
He defined depression (or melancholy) as "a state of mind in which
a man is so out of touch with his environment that life has lost its
sweetness." [70] Osler probably learned to use the more mature
defenses in his family of origin, but he also absorbed them from
the mentors, both living and historical, that he cultivated along the
way. He understood that we can absorb such defenses from the
great minds of the ages, and it was partly for this reason that he
advised daily contact with "the saints of humanity"—the biblical
writers, the Stoic philosophers, Cervantes, Shakespeare, Sir
Thomas Browne, and many others. He understood that such reading can have a powerful if subliminal impact:

> For the student of medicine the writings of Sir Thomas Browne
> have a very positive value. The charm of high thoughts clad in
> beautiful language may win some readers to a love of good litera-
> ture; but beyond this there is a still greater advantage. Like the
> "Thoughts of Marcus Aurelius" and the "Enchiridion" of Epictetus,
> the "Religio" is full of counsels of perfection which appeal to the
> mind of youth, still plastic and unhardened by contact with the
> world. Carefully studied, from such books come subtle influences
> which give stability to character and help to give a man a sane
> outlook on the complex problems of life. [71]

Indeed, Sir Thomas Browne wrote of the importance of avoiding at all costs the kind of free-floating anger and hostility that bring on heart attacks:

> Let not the Sun in Capricorn [that is, even when the days are shortest] go down upon thy wrath, but write thy wrongs in Ashes. Draw the Curtain of night upon injuries, shut them up in the Tower of Oblivion and let them be as though they had not been. To forgive our Enemies, yet hope that God will punish them, is not to forgive enough. To forgive them ourselves, and not to pray God to forgive them, is a partial piece of Charity. Forgive thine enemies totally, and without any reserve that however God will revenge thee.[72]

Browne also noted that revenge is to be discouraged for it is likely to backfire: "Let thy Arrows of Revenge fly short, or be aimed like those of *Jonathan*, to fall beside the mark." [73] In *Don Quixote*, Cervantes similarly showed that negative emotions become the enemy within us:

> Our greatest Foes, and whom we must chiefly combat, are within. Envy we must overcome by Generosity and Nobleness of Soul; Anger, by a repos'd and easy Mind; Riot and Drowsiness, by Vigilance and Temperance; Lasciviousness, by our inviolable Fidelity to those who are Mistresses of our Thoughts; and Sloth, by our indefatigable Peregrinations through the Universe.[74]

Indeed, Cervantes's novel is a classic demonstration of the usefulness of altruism, anticipation, sublimation, and humor as defenses against stress.

Osler knew that life contains few guarantees, that disappointment and failure can ensue from even our best efforts. As he told students, Stoic philosophy helps a great deal:

> It is sad to think that, for some of you, there is in store disappointment, perhaps failure. You cannot hope, of course, to escape from the cares and anxieties incident to professional life. Stand up bravely, even against the worst. . . . Well for you, if you wrestle on, for in persistency lies victory, and with the morning may come the wished-for blessing. But not always; there is a struggle with defeat which some of you will have to bear, and it will be well for you in that day to have cultivated a cheerful equanimity.[75]

How successful was Osler at using the more mature defense mechanisms? The evidence suggests that he frequently relied on sublimation, altruism, anticipation, and humor (see Chapters 1 and 6). His biographer Edith Reid noted:

> With Dr. Osler the rational and emotional life were both convincing, both genuine—it was impossible for him to be either sentimental or irrational. His intellect was entirely truthful and he found truth often in the most unpromising places; but he left a broad margin for the opinion of others and to rectify mistakes.[76]

These observations accord with many others made of Osler at different points of his life by various observers. But he was not blind to the negative emotions around him, and knew what it is like to be resented. When Osler arrived in Philadelphia from Montreal in 1884, seeds of resentment had already been planted. Selecting a worthy successor to the famous William Pepper was a matter of wide concern throughout the University of Pennsylvania. Many people were disappointed that the job had been given to a young Canadian. Osler ignored the resentment and got on with his work. One colleague recalled that "Osler's pervasive enthusiasm and his imperturbable friendliness, agreeably punctuated with his mischievous whimsies, soon won him the affection of his colleagues and the respect of the Philadelphia profession at large." [77] He knew the importance of not worrying too much about what others think. He wrote in an obituary of a colleague who was apparently humorless:

> Upon men obviously striving to be taken at their own valuation the world has no mercy; now and again one wins out, but the majority form a battered band whose work and worth never receive a due mead of appreciation. It is the careless sinner who goes a-whistling and working through life, caring not for what the world thinks, who gets more than his due.[78]

Osler's ability to use the mature defense mechanisms was severely tested by his son's death in World War I (see Chapter 8). Less than a week after Revere was killed, he was back visiting hospitals and working on his textbook—again illustrating anticipation, sublimation, and altruism. As he later confided,

> Grief is a hard companion, particularly to an optimist, & to one who has been a stranger to it for so many years. We decided to keep the

flag flying & let no outward action demonstrate, if possible, the aching hearts.[79]

In these painful sentences, Osler summed up his philosophy of positive thinking, of keeping the flag high however harsh the wind. And when the war ended he did not speak of retribution but instead looked forward to the possibility of world peace.

5

LEARN

AND

TEACH

Driving Plato's Horses

Osler defined himself mainly as an educator. He loved the learning process and regarded his students as fellow learners. He popularized teaching medicine at the bedside and said that he wanted no epitaph other than that he had taught medical students in the wards. He championed continuing medical education and stricter licensing standards for physicians. Yet his commitment to education transcended the hospital and clinic environments. He was a university person in the broad sense of belonging to a worldwide community of scholars. When he dedicated the *Aequanimitas* collection of essays to Daniel Coit Gilman "in memory of those happy days in 1889 when, under your guidance, the Johns Hopkins Hospital was organized and opened; and in grateful recognition of your active and intelligent interest in medical education," he was acknowledging that Gilman, as president of The Johns Hopkins University, had embraced the medical school in spirit as well as name. It is in the context of education that we find many of Osler's loftiest messages.

VALUE EDUCATION

Education ranked high among Osler's unifying principles (see Chapter 1). He thought about the definition of education and asked rhetorically:

> What, after all, is education but a subtle, slowly-affected change, due to the action upon us of the Externals; of the written record of the great minds of all ages, of the beautiful and harmonious surroundings of nature and of art, and of the lives, good or ill, of our fellows—these alone educate us, these alone mould the developing minds.[1]

He urged young people to cherish "the student life" as a special time:

> Learn to love the freedom of the student life, only too quickly to pass away; the absence of the coarser cares of after days, the joy in comradeship, the delight in new work, the happiness in knowing that you are making progress. Once only can you enjoy these pleasures.[2]

Osler held that poorly educated physicians are a menace to society:

> A man cannot become a competent surgeon without a full knowledge of human anatomy and physiology, and the physician without physiology and chemistry flounders along in an aimless fashion, never able to gain any accurate conception of disease, practising a sort of popgun pharmacy, hitting now the malady and again the patient, he himself not knowing which.[3]

And he stressed lifelong learning:

> If the license to practise meant the completion of his education how sad it would be for the practitioner, how distressing to his patients! More clearly than any other the physician should illustrate the truth of Plato's saying that education is a life-long process.[4]

His own ability to keep up was almost legendary. A student marveled that Osler "could read and digest medical literature more rapidly than anyone I have ever met." [5]

Osler kept up not only with medicine and science but also with the humanities to the extent that he could hold his own with professors of English, history, philosophy, and the classics. He treasured universities especially for their productive scholars:

> The great possession of any University is its great names. It is not the "pride, pomp and circumstance" of an institution which bring honour, nor its wealth, nor the number of its schools, not the students who throng its halls, but the *men* who have trodden in its service the thorny road through toil, even through hate, to the serene abode of Fame, climbing "like stars to their appointed height." These bring glory, and it should thrill the heart of every alumnus. [6]

The goals of a university should be simply "to teach and to think." [7] At 61, Osler expanded on these functions:

> All are agreed that a university has a dual function—to learn and to advance learning. I use the word "learn" in the old sense—met with in the Bible and still used colloquially—as it expresses the mental attitude of the student towards his Alma Mater, *"totius litteratorii studii altrix prima* [the chief nurse of the study of every schoolteacher]." In mind, manners and morals the young man seeks life's equipment when he says to his Alma Mater in the words of the Psalmist, "O learn me true understanding and knowledge." To learn the use of his mind, to learn good manners, and to learn to drive Plato's horses, form the marrow of an education within the reach of every citizen, but to which universities minister in a very special way; and it should be comprehensive, fitting a man, in Milton's words, "to perform all the offices, private and public, of peace or of war." The other great function of a university is to advance learning, to increase man's knowledge of man and of nature. [8]

This dual function of universities demanded that faculty be recruited who could add to the world's body of knowledge as well as teach:

> In a school which . . . wishes to do thinking as well as teaching, men must be selected who are not only thoroughly *au courant* with the best work in their department the world over, but who also have ideas, with ambition and energy to put them into force—men who

can add each one in his sphere, to the store of the world's knowledge.[9]

Osler recognized that teaching and research are different skills
that do not necessarily go hand in hand. He held that teachers
must have three essential qualities: knowledge, enthusiasm, and

> a *sense of obligation*, that feeling which impels a teacher to be also
> a contributor, and to add to the stores from which he so freely
> draws. And precisely here is the necessity to know the best that is
> taught in this branch, the world over. The investigator, to be suc-
> cessful, must start abreast of the knowledge of the day, and he
> differs from the teacher, who, living in the present, expounds only
> what is current, in that his thoughts must be in the future, and his
> ways and work in advance of the day in which he lives.[10]

Skilled researchers can fail as teachers:

> Teachers who teach current knowledge are not necessarily investiga-
> tors; many have not had the needful training; others have not the
> needful time. The very best instructor for students may have no con-
> ception of the higher lines of work in his branch, and contrariwise,
> how many brilliant investigators have been wretched teachers?[11]

Osler praised American colleges and universities for seeking out
the best teachers from all parts of the world:

> It is gratifying to note the broad liberality displayed by American
> colleges in welcoming from all parts teachers who may have shown
> any special fitness, emulating in this respect the liberality of the
> Athenians, in whose porticoes and lecture halls the stranger was
> greeted as a citizen and judged by his mental gifts alone.[12]

Just as teachers must be committed to their students, so should
students value their teachers:

> What, for example, is more proper than the pride which we feel in
> our teachers, in the university from which we have graduated, in the
> hospital at which we have been trained? He is a "poor sort" who is
> free from such feelings, which only manifest a proper loyalty.[13]

Holding that "the greatness of a school lies in brains not bricks," [14]
Osler considered educators to be among society's most valuable
members.

Next to its faculty, the university's most important asset was its
books: "Books are the tools of the mind, and in a community of

progressive scholars the literature of the world in the different departments of knowledge must be represented." [15] One of Osler's most frequently quoted remarks went:

> It is hard for me to speak of the value of libraries in terms which would not seem exaggerated. Books have been my delight these thirty years, and from them I have received incalculable benefits. To study the phenomena of disease without books is to sail an uncharted sea, while to study books without patients is not to go to sea at all. Only a maker of books can appreciate the labours of others at their true value.

He continued:

> For the teacher and the worker a great library . . . is indispensable. They must know the world's best work and know it at once. They mint and make current coin the ore so widely scattered in journals, transactions, and monographs.

All physicians—and especially those in the field, remote from universities—should cherish their personal libraries:

> For the general practitioner a well-used library is one of the few correctives of the premature senility which is so apt to overtake him. Self-centred, self-taught, he leads a solitary life, and unless his every-day experience is controlled by careful reading or by the attrition of a medical society it soon ceases to be of the slightest value and becomes a mere accretion of isolated facts, without correlation. It is astonishing with how little reading a doctor can practise medicine, but it is not astonishing how badly he may do it. [16]

One of his unfinished papers was entitled "The College of the Book," in which he dealt with bookmaking from start to finish. [17] Books and libraries thus symbolized his commitment to education and the learning process.

OBSERVE AND THINK

Osler approached medicine mainly as a naturalist rather than as an experimentalist, which is to say that his basic method was to observe and reason rather than to analyze a single variable under controlled conditions. He concentrated especially on anatomic pathology, seeking to correlate structure with function in health and disease. The naturalist's approach requires critical thinking; as Osler put it, "That man can interrogate as well as observe nature was a lesson slowly learned in his evolution." [18] Osler credited the Greeks, especially the Hippocratic writers, for insisting that medicine should be based on descriptive observation rather than on religion or magic:

> Everywhere one finds a strong, clear common sense, which refuses to be entangled either in theological or philosophical speculations. . . . Empiricism, experience, the collection of facts, the evidence of the senses, the avoidance of philosophical speculations, were the distinguishing features of Hippocratic medicine. [19]

Observation must be combined with thinking:

> Observation *plus* thinking has given us the vast stores of knowledge we now possess of the structure of the bodies of living creatures in health and disease. There have been two inherent difficulties—to get men to see straight and to get men to think clearly; but in spite of the frailty of the instrument, the method has been one of the most powerful ever placed in the hands of man. [20]

From these premises followed a straightforward philosophy of teaching: "Teach [the student] how to observe, give him plenty of facts to observe and the lessons will come out of the facts themselves." [21] Indeed,

> The whole art of medicine is in observation, as the old motto goes, but to educate the eye to see, the ear to hear and the finger to feel takes time, and to make a beginning, to start a man on the right path, is all that we can do. We expect too much of the student and we try to teach him too much. Give him good methods and a proper point of view, and all other things will be added, as his experience grows. [22]

He urged young physicians never to tire of observation:

> Note with accuracy and care everything that comes within your professional ken. . . . Let nothing slip by you; the ordinary humdrum cases of the morning routine may have been accurately described and pictured, but study each one separately as though it were new—so it is so far as your special experience goes; and if the spirit of the student is in you the lesson will be there. [23]

He admired the great physicians of the past for their powers of observation. Thus "Sydenham's chief merit is that he taught the profession to return to Hippocratic methods of careful observation and study";[24] Locke was a "keen observer, a constant note-taker, and of most neat and accurate literary habits";[25]and the great French clinician Louis was "a voluminous note-taker . . . [who] collected in this time an enormous number of important facts." [26] But he understood that to be of value, observation must be combined with thinking and asking questions.

Osler combined observation with reasoning according to what has been called the method of Zadig. Zadig, the hero of a 1747 novelette by Voltaire, was a wealthy young Babylonian with an astounding ability to find truth by reasoning from seemingly trivial facts. For example, from the footprints of the queen's dog, which he had never seen, he induced that the animal was a small, long-eared, slightly lame female that had given birth a few days earlier.[27] Osler advised his students that they, like Zadig, should bring to the bedside the detective's ability to make deductions or inferences from inconspicuous features:

> The value of experience is not in seeing much, but in seeing wisely. Experience in the true sense of the term does not come to all with years or with increasing opportunities. Growth in the acquisition of facts is not necessarily associated with development. . . . The growth which is organic and enduring, is totally different, marked by changes of an unmistakable character. The observations are made with accuracy and care, no pains are spared, nothing is thought a trouble in the investigation of a problem. . . . Insensibly, year by year, a man finds that there has been in his mental protoplasm not only growth by assimilation but an actual development, bringing fuller powers of observation, additional capabilities of mental nutrition, and that increased breadth of view which is of the very essence of wisdom.[28]

A student recalled Osler's point that "the diagnosis of a patient's disease often stared one in the face, if one possesses a 'seeing eye,' has good light, and possesses proper reasoning powers." [29] He held that the ability to reason could be developed through practice and experience.

Osler's clinical experience began and continued with anatomic pathology. The pathologist William G. MacCallum remarked that "no clinician in English-speaking countries has had at his command such a wide and detailed knowledge of morbid anatomy as Osler." He not only made careful observations about cases but also saw "the usefulness of considering together a group or series of similar cases." MacCallum held that Osler's "clearness of vision with regard to the actual natural history of disease, always referring to a well-remembered series of cases, helped to make his teaching a memorable delight to his students." [30] Osler wrote:

> I am firmly convinced that the best book in medicine is the book of Nature, as written large in the bodies of men. You remember the answer of the immortal Hunter, when asked what books the student should read in anatomy—he opened the door of the dissecting-room and pointed to the tables. Erasmus further adds that the most important thing is not how much you know, but the quality of what you know. [31]

Osler developed an exceptional "ability to look beyond the gross and even the detail of pathological lesions, and apply them to the living." [32] Against this background, his curriculum for medical students was straightforward. They should learn progressively how to observe and how to reason: "The work consists in, first, the training of the senses in the observation of disease; secondly, courses in physical diagnosis and clinical microscopy; and, thirdly, practical work in history taking, fourthly, the general medical clinic in the amphitheater." [33] The essentials were a notebook, a library, and—after graduation—periodic refresher courses:

> Given the sacred hunger and proper preliminary training, the student-practitioner requires at least three things with which to stimulate and maintain his education, a notebook, a library, and a quinquennial braindusting. I wish I had time to speak of the value of note-taking. You can do nothing as a student in practice without it. Carry a small notebook which will fit into your waistcoat pocket, and never ask a new patient a question without notebook and pencil in hand. After the examination of a pneumonia case two minutes will suffice to record the essentials in the daily progress. Routine and system when once made a habit, facilitate work, and the busier you are the more time you will have to make observations after examining a patient. Jot a comment at the end of the notes: "clear case," "case illustrating obscurity of symptoms," "error in diagnosis," etc. . . . The study of the cases, the relation they bear to each other and to the cases in literature—here comes in the difficulty.

Begin early to make a threefold category—clear cases, doubtful cases, mistakes. And learn to play the game fair, no self-deception, no shrinking from the truth; mercy and consideration for the other man, but none for yourself, upon whom you have to keep an incessant watch. You remember Lincoln's famous *mot* about the impossibility of fooling all of the people all of the time. It does not hold good for the individual who can fool himself to his heart's content all of the time.[34]

Osler was a "notebook man." He told students, "Don't trust your memory. Make notes. Write down your observations." [35] He usually read with a pen in his right hand and would jot down notes as he went along. In his later years, he often wrote fragmentary comments that he placed in books, many of which still exist in his library.[36] He exhorted young physicians:

In a ten or fifteen years' service, travelling with seeing eyes and hearing ears, and carefully kept note-books, just think what a storehouse of clinical material may be at the command of any one of you—material not only valuable in itself to the profession, but of infinite value to you personally in its acquisition, rendering you painstaking and accurate, and giving you, year by year, an increasing experience.[37]

Not only should observations lead to questions, but—and perhaps more importantly—questions should lead to observations. Osler thus lauded two students:

The Hunterian "Do not think, but try" attitude of mind is the important one to cultivate. The question came up one day, when discussing the grooves left on the nails after fever, how long it took for the nail to grow out, from root to edge. A majority of the class had no further interest; a few looked it up in books; two men marked their nails at the root with nitrate of silver, and a few months later had positive knowledge on the subject. They showed the proper spirit.[38]

Stimulated by this remark of Osler's, the late Dr. William B. Bean studied the growth of his left thumbnail throughout his adult life. He determined that the growth rate of his left thumbnail correlated with the stresses of his life and with aging, a "natural kymograph"—an observation with which Osler no doubt would have been pleased.[39]

William Sydney Thayer paraphrased bedside aphorisms gleaned from his long association with Osler at Johns Hopkins:

Observe, record, tabulate, communicate.

Use your five senses. The art of the practice of medicine is to be learned only by experience; 'tis not an inheritance; it cannot be revealed. Learn to see, learn to hear, learn to feel, learn to smell, and know that by practice alone can you become expert. Medicine is learned by the bedside and not in the classroom. Let not your conceptions of the manifestations of disease come from words heard in the lecture room or read from the book. See, and then reason and compare and control. But see first. No two eyes see the same thing. No two mirrors give forth the same reflection. Let your word be your slave and not your master.

Live in the ward. Do not waste the hours of daylight in listening to that which you may read by night. But when you have seen, read. And when you can, read the original descriptions of the masters who, with crude methods of study, saw so clearly.

Record that which you have seen; make a note at the time; do not wait. "The flighty purpose never is o'ertook, unless the deed go with it."

Memory plays strange pranks with facts. The rocks and fissures and gullies of the mountain-side melt quickly into the smooth, blue outlines of the distant panorama. Viewed through the perspective of memory, an unrecorded observation, the vital details long since lost, easily changes its countenance and sinks obediently into the frame fashioned by the fancy of the moment.

Always note and record the unusual. Keep and compare your observations. Communicate or publish short notes on anything that is striking or new. Do not waste your time in compilations, but when your observations are sufficient, do not let them die with you. Study them, tabulate them, seek the points of contact which may reveal the underlying law. Some things can be learned only by statistical comparison. If you have the good fortune to command a large clinic, remember that one of your chief duties is the tabulation and analysis of the carefully recorded experience.[40]

Osler sometimes summarized his method of teaching by saying, "We take as our motto the old maxim: 'The whole art of medicine is in observation.' "[41] Thayer's paraphrasing indicates, however, a broader appreciation of learning theory as understood today—an

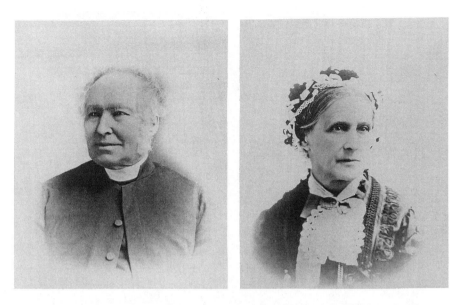

William Osler's parents, Featherstone Lake Osler (1805–1895) and Ellen Free Pickton Osler (1806–1907).

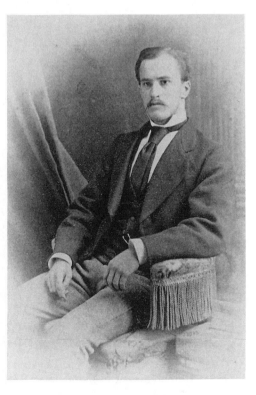

Osler as a young man. After graduating from McGill Medical School, Montreal, in 1872, he studied in Europe for two years and then returned to McGill in 1874 as instructor in medicine.

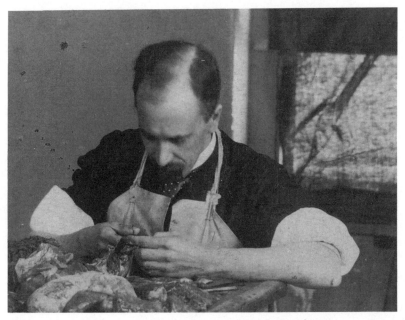

Osler performing an autopsy at Blockley Hospital, Philadelphia, circa 1886–1889. His experience in pathology at McGill and at the University of Pennsylvania formed the basis for his becoming a consummate diagnostician.

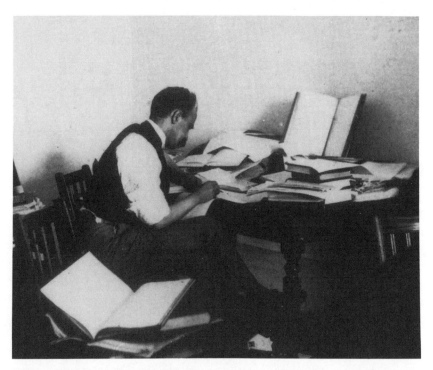

Osler at work on his textbook, *The Principles and Practice of Medicine*, in 1891. He had moved to Baltimore in 1889 to be Chair of Medicine at the new medical school at Johns Hopkins, but the school had not yet opened—affording him time to write the book that made him famous throughout much of the world.

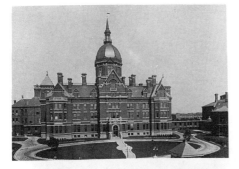

The administration building of The Johns Hopkins Hospital, circa 1892. The building provided quarters for the resident physicians. Osler wrote most of his textbook in the study of one of the obstetrical residents, Dr. Hunter Robb.

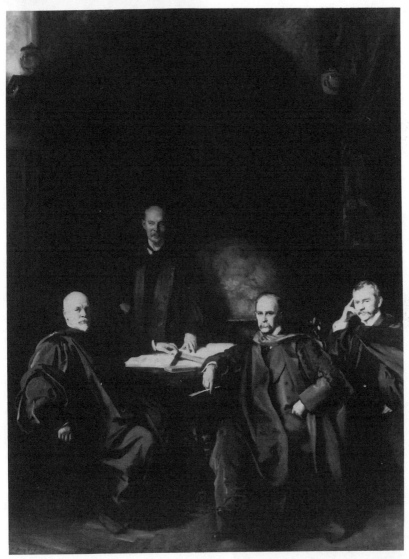

"The Four Doctors," painted by John Singer Sargent in 1905, honored the famous chiefs of service associated with the founding of the Johns Hopkins University School of Medicine. From left are pathologist William H. Welch, surgeon William S. Halsted, Osler, and gynecologist Howard A. Kelly. Sargent is said to have remarked of Osler that he had never before painted a man with an olive-green complexion.

William and Grace Osler in 1894.
They were married in 1892 after a
courtship the details of which are
largely unknown. She was the
great-granddaughter of the American Revolutionary patriot Paul Revere, and the widow of a Philadelphia surgeon, Dr. Samuel W. Gross.

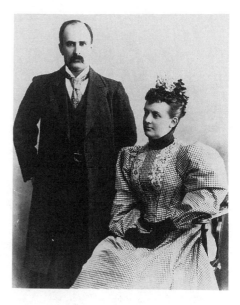

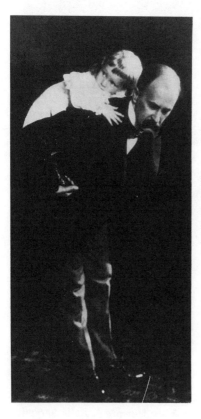

Edward Revere Osler was born December
28, 1895. The Oslers—being an older couple and having lost their first child—were
ecstatic. On this photograph Osler wrote,
"And on his shoulders, not a lamb, a Kid!"

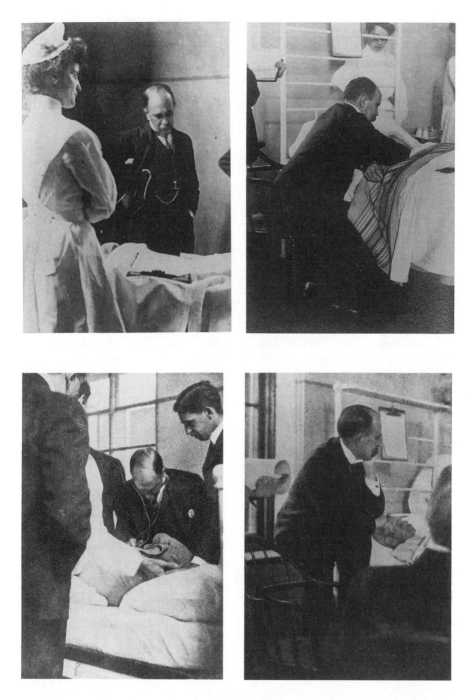

Osler at the bedside, circa 1903. These snapshots, taken by Dr. T. W. Clarke on Ward F of The Johns Hopkins Hospital, have been labeled (clockwise, from upper left) "Viewing the charts," "Palpation," "Contemplation," and "Auscultation."

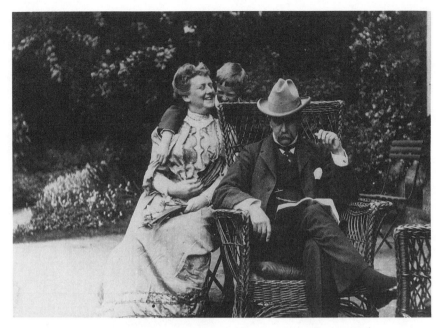

Grace, Revere, and William Osler at Oxford, June 1905, after Osler had become Regius Professor of Medicine. Revere was ten years old.

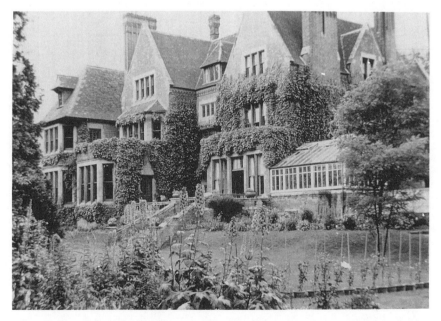

The Osler home at 13 Norham Gardens, Oxford, was widely known as "The Open Arms," a mecca for visitors from North America.

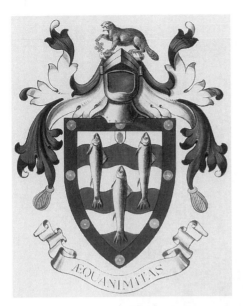

Knighted in 1911, Osler took "aequanimitas" (equanimity; calmness) as the motto for his coat of arms. The beaver symbolizes his native Canada; the fish were a tribute to his son, Revere, an ardent angler.

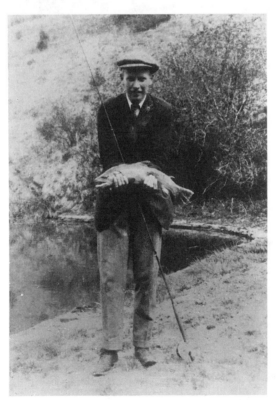

Revere Osler with a record trout caught in May, 1917, while on leave from the army. Osler had nicknamed his son "Isaac" after Izaac Walton, the great angler.

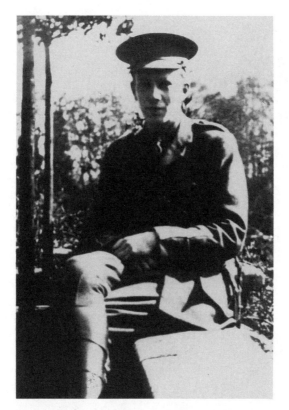

Second Lieutenant Revere Osler in uniform, World War I. William and Grace Osler supported the British war effort despite concerns about their only surviving son's presence on the front lines.

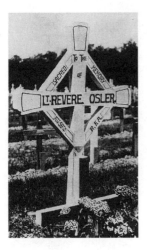

On August 30, 1917, Revere Osler died of wounds from artillery fire in Belgium and was buried there.

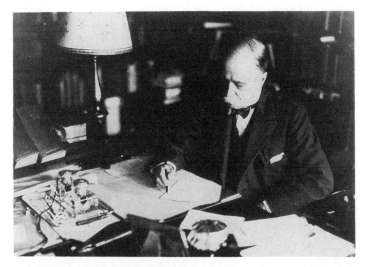

Osler at his desk at Oxford. In his last years Osler worked on cataloging his books as the *Bibliotheca Osleriana*.

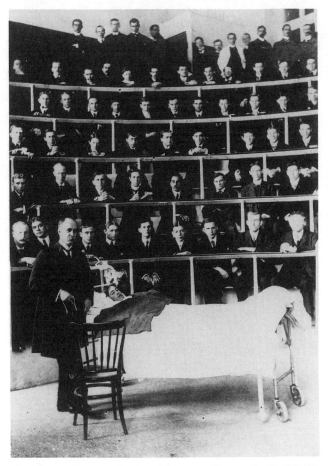

Osler conducting a clinic at the Royal Victoria Hospital, McGill University, Montreal, in 1906. He had come to Canada from England for the celebration of his mother's 100th birthday.

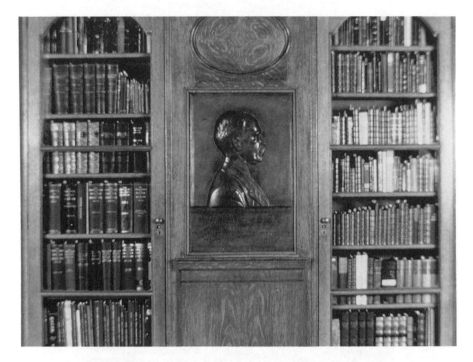

The Osler niche at the Osler Library of the History of Medicine, McGill University, Montreal. Osler's relief—known as the Vernon plaque—is flanked on the left by his own writings and on the right by his collection of the works of Sir Thomas Browne, the seventeenth-century English physician whom Osler called his "lifelong mentor." Behind the panel just below the plaque rest the ashes of Sir William and Lady Osler.

ongoing cycle of observation, reflection, generalization, and refinement by further experience.

COMBINE PRINCIPLES AND PRACTICE

Much as he valued universities for their famous professors, fine books, and additions to the sum of knowledge, Osler held that the main goal of medical schools was to turn out effective doctors. He lived at a time when specialization was becoming rampant in medicine as in other fields. However, he championed the cause of family physicians. Thus he observed to the members of the Canadian Medical Association:

> It is amusing to read and hear of the passing of the family physician. There never was a time in our history in which he was so much in evidence. . . . He is the standard by which we are measured. What he is, we are; and the estimate of the profession in the eyes of the public is their estimate of him. A well-trained, sensible doctor is one of the most valuable assets of a community, worth to-day, as in Homer's time, many another man. To make him efficient is our highest ambition as teachers, to save him from evil should be our constant care as a guild.[42]

He went on to quote Sir Thomas Browne to the effect that actions speak louder than words:

> But as Sir Thomas Browne—most liberal of men and most distinguished of general practitioners—so beautifully remarks: "These are Thoughts of things which Thoughts but tenderly touch," and it may be sufficient to remind this audience, made up of practical men, *that the word of action is stronger than the word of speech.*[43]

He urged, "To be of any value an education should prepare for life's work." [44] And he stressed principles: "Some of you may have heard of the lecture-room motto of that distinguished pathologist and surgeon, and the first systematic writer on morbid anatomy in the United States, S. D. Gross, "Principles, gentlemen, principles! Principles!!" [45] This dual emphasis was implicit in the title of his textbook: *The Principles and Practice of Medicine.*

Osler told medical students to study people as well as books. He feared that "common sense in matters medical is rare, and is usually in inverse ratio to the degree of education." [46] He therefore urged students:

> Divide your attentions equally between books and men. The strength of the student of books is to sit still—two or three hours at a stretch—eating the heart out of a subject with pencil and note-book in hand, determined to master the details and intricacies, focussing all your energies on its difficulties. Get accustomed to test all sorts of book problems and statements for yourself, and take as little as possible on trust.[47]

Failure to study people as well as books can spell disaster:

> Curiously enough, the student-practitioner may find studiousness to be a stumbling-block in his career. A bookish man may never succeed; deep-versed in books, he may not be able to use his knowledge to practical effect, or, more likely, his failure is not because he has studied books much, but because he has not studied men more.[48]

Acknowledging that most graduates would be clinicians rather than researchers, he held that medical education must be practical as well as theoretical: "The problem before us as teachers may be very briefly stated: to give to our students an education of such a character that they can become sensible practitioners—the destiny of seven-eighths of them." [49]

Osler went so far as to say, "the greatest difficulty in life is to make knowledge effective, to convert it into practical wisdom." [50] He made it clear that knowledge and practical wisdom can be different commodities:

> No one ever drew a more skilful distinction than Cowper in his oft-quoted lines, which I am never tired of repeating in a medical audience:
>
> > Knowledge and wisdom, far from being one,
> > Have oft-times no connexion. Knowledge dwells
> > In heads replete with thoughts of other men;
> > Wisdom in minds attentive to their own.
> > Knowledge is proud that he has learned so much;
> > Wisdom is humble that he knows no more.

What we call sense or wisdom is knowledge, ready for use, made effective, and bears the same relation to knowledge itself that bread does to wheat. . . . One of the most delightful sayings of antiquity is the remark of Heraclitus upon his predecessors—that they had much knowledge but no sense—which indicates that the noble old Ephesian had a keen appreciation of their difference; and the distinction, too, is well drawn by Tennyson in the oft-quoted line:

Knowledge comes but wisdom lingers.[51]

These considerations raise an issue: What is the best kind of clinical teacher? A practicing doctor who spends most of his time seeing patients or a researcher who augments the knowledge base?

Even in his prime at Johns Hopkins, Osler was what would be considered today a part-time clinical teacher. At that time, nearly all clinical faculty members did a great deal of private practice. Osler spent most mornings teaching at the hospital and clinic but, after 1892, began to spend his afternoons mainly in a private consulting practice carried out largely at his home. His practice was successful, indeed too successful as it robbed him of time for his cherished academic pursuits.[52] In part because of Osler's influence, however, full-time clinical teachers came to be the norm at most medical schools. The attention given to Osler's textbook by Rockefeller advisor Frederick T. Gates eventually led to large Rockefeller grants to fund clinical professorships. Osler, who was by that time at Oxford, deplored the notion that medical students might be taught by physicians who did not take care of patients:

The burning question to be settled by this generation relates to the whole-time clinical teacher. It has been forced on the profession by men who know nothing of clinical medicine, and there has been a "mess of pottage" side to the business in the shape of big Rockefeller cheques at which my gorge rises. To have a group of cloistered clinicians away completely from the broad current of professional life would be bad for teacher and worse for student. The primary work of a professor of medicine in a medical school is in the wards, teaching his pupils how to deal with patients and their diseases. His business is to turn out men who know how to handle the sick. His business, also, is to bring into play all the resources of the laboratories in the investigation of disease.[53]

He believed that full-time clinical faculty appointments would lead to less emphasis on teaching and more emphasis on research. After World War II, large infusions of government monies led to rapid growth of full-time clinical faculties at most American medical schools. Osler's prophecy that teaching would take a back seat to research in the academic reward system came true, and the issue of full-time versus part-time clinical teachers continues to be debated.[54]

BE INTELLECTUALLY HONEST

Like all good academicians, Osler knew that intellectual honesty is a precious commodity that must be constantly safeguarded. His writings suggest at least four components: humility, skepticism, acknowledgment of the limits of truth, and the ability to tolerate the anxiety of uncertainty.

In 1899 Osler reminisced that in the 25 years since he had first joined the faculty at McGill, "I have learned . . . to be a better student, and to be ready to say to my fellow students 'I do not know.' " [55] He gave a more complete statement concerning humility while speaking at the University of Minnesota:

> In these days of aggressive self-assertion, when the stress of competition is so keen and the desire to make the most of oneself so universal, it may seem a little old-fashioned to preach the necessity of this virtue, but I insist for its own sake, and for the sake of what it brings, that a due humility should take the place of honour on the list [of virtues for physicians]. For its own sake, since with it comes not only a reverence for truth, but also a proper estimation of the difficulties encountered in our search for it. More perhaps than any other professional, the doctor has a curious—shall I say morbid?—sensitiveness to (what he regards) personal error. In a way this is right; but it is too often accompanied by a *cocksureness* of opinion which, if encouraged, leads him to so lively a conceit that the mere suggestion of mistake under any circumstances is regarded as a reflection on his honour, a reflection equally resented whether of lay or of professional origin. Start out with the conviction that absolute truth is hard to reach in matters relating to our fellow creatures, healthy or diseased, that slips in observation are inevitable even with the best trained faculties, that errors in judgment must occur in the practice of an art which consists largely of

balancing probabilities;—start, I say, with this attitude in mind, and mistakes will be acknowledged and regretted; but instead of a slow process of self-deception, with ever increasing inability to recognize truth, you will draw from your errors the very lessons which may enable you to avoid their repetition.

And, for the sake of what it brings, this grace of humility is a precious gift. When to the sessions of sweet silent thought you summon up the remembrance of your own imperfections, the faults of your brothers will seem less grievous, and, in the quaint language of Sir Thomas Browne, you will "allow one eye for what is laudable in them." [56]

Humility thus requires openness to the possibility of error. In 1893 Osler concluded a series of lectures on the diagnosis of abdominal tumors by remembering one of his teachers in Berlin,

> that true Asclepiad, Ludwig Traube, who, adding *probity* to learning, sagacity, and humanity, reached the full stature of the Hippocratean physician. When acknowledging some error he would say—often in a soft, meditative manner, as if gently reproaching himself—Have we carefully observed all the facts of the case? Yes. Did the art permit of a judgment on the facts under consideration? Yes. Did we reason correctly upon the data before us? No. *Wir haben nicht richtig gedacht* [We did not think correctly].[57]

Even Osler sometimes forgot that in searching for truth we should restrain our pride. Once, for example, he put his ego on the line over whether a heart lesion was congenital or acquired and, shown wrong, hurried out of the autopsy room, coattails flying.[58] But such instances aside, he practiced intellectual honesty based on a healthy skepticism.

Osler's skepticism can be traced at least in part to the influence of Sir Thomas Browne, whose views merit a brief review. Browne praised the skeptical philosophers of ancient Greece:

> I have run through all sects, yet find no rest in any; though our first studies and *junior* endeavors may style us Peripatetics, Stoics, or Academics, yet I perceive the wisest heads prove at last almost all Skeptics, and stand like *Janus* in the field of knowledge.[59]

He acknowledged that

> we are often constrained to stand alone against the strength of opinion; and to meet the Goliath and Giant of Authority, with

contemptible pibbles, and feeble arguments, drawn from the scrip and slender stock of our selves.[60]

And we are vulnerable to deception, for

a cause of common Errors is the Credulity of men, that is, an easy assent to what is obtruded, or a believing at first ear what is delivered by others.[61]

Browne, who pondered at length such arcane issues as why artists painted navels on Adam and Eve, recognized that

a man may be in as just possession of Truth as of a City, and yet be forced to surrender; 'tis therefore far better to enjoy her with peace, then to hazzard her on a battle.[62]

However, in the end, we must refuse to bow down before authority, since

the most mortal enemy unto knowledge, and that which has done the greatest execution upon truth, has been a peremptory adhesion unto Authority, and more especially the establishing of our belief upon the dictates of Antiquity.[63]

As an avowed protégé of Browne, Osler was well known as a skeptic not only of the drugs available to him but also of new theories.

Indeed, he was skeptical toward medical knowledge in general. He admired the questioning attitude that arose especially in Paris during the early years of the nineteenth century, the place and time that gave rise to statistics in medical research. According to Osler, American students who studied there, such as Boston's Oliver Wendell Holmes and Rhode Island's Elisha Bartlett, "probably acquired in Paris three principles: 'Not to take authority when I can have facts; not to guess when I can know; not to think a man must take physic because he is sick.' " [64] Perhaps it was because of his skeptical attitude that Osler was not always on the cutting edge of major medical knowledge. MacCallum recalled that Osler had "shown himself critical and sane and quite unwilling to pursue what seemed a fantastic theory unless convinced by definite proofs." [65] He hesitated before accepting some of the implications of the germ theory of disease. He does not seem to have grasped right away the significance of the breakthroughs made by Joseph Lister (antisepsis in surgery), Robert Koch (a bacillus as the cause of tuberculosis), or Alphonse Laveran (parasites as the cause of malaria). He held that healthy skepticism is the best course especially for those on the front lines of medical practice:

> The salt of life for him [the family physician] is a judicious scepticism, not the coarse, crude form, but the sober sense of honest doubt expressed in the maxim of the sly old Sicilian Epicharmus, "Be sober and distrustful; these are the sinews of the understanding." A great advantage, too, of a sceptical attitude of mind is, as Green the historian remarks, "One is never very surprised or angry to find that one's opponents are in the right." [66]

Osler suggested that skepticism applies not only to scientific matters but also to everyday life. He urged caution especially regarding the news media: "Believe nothing that you see in the newspapers. . . . If you see anything in them that you know is true, begin to doubt it at once." [67] But he was also skeptical in the broader sense, recognizing that "truth" is often a will-o'-the-wisp abstraction.

Each generation, Osler maintained, must be willing to challenge even the most basic assumptions: "Truth has been well called the daughter of Time, and even in anatomy, which is a science in a state of fact, the point of view changes with successive generations." [68] In one of his farewell addresses to North American medical students in 1905, Osler exhorted them:

> At the outset do not be worried about this big question—Truth. It is a very simple matter if each one of you starts with the desire to get as much as possible. No human being is constituted to know the truth, the whole truth, and nothing but the truth; and even the best of men must be content with fragments, with partial glimpses, never the full fruition. . . . The truth is the best you can get with your best endeavour, the best that the best men accept—with this you must learn to be satisfied, retaining at the same time with due humility an earnest desire for an ever larger portion.[69]

In medicine especially, truth can best be regarded as a matter of probability: "Probability is the rule of life—especially under the skin. Never make a positive diagnosis." [70] Similarly,

> Variability is the law of life, and as no two faces are the same, so no two bodies are alike, and no two individuals react alike and behave alike under the abnormal conditions which we know as disease. This is the fundamental difficulty in the education of the physician,

and one which he may never grasp, or he takes it so tenderly that it hurts instead of boldly accepting the axiom of Bishop Butler, more true of medicine than of any other profession: "Probability is the guide of life." Surrounded by people who demand certainty, and not philosopher enough to agree with Locke that "*Probability supplies the defect of our knowledge and guides us when that fails and is always conversant about things of which we have no certainty,*" the practitioner too often gets into the habit of mind which resents the thought that opinion, not full knowledge, must be his stay and prop.[71]

To be sure, Osler acknowledged that on occasion one can be certain, as when a particular finding is diagnostic: "Although one swallow does not make a summer, one tophus makes gout and one crescent malaria." [72] However, his dominant attitude was that of a truth-searching skeptic or—in today's parlance—a critical thinker.[73]

And finally, Osler fully acknowledged that medical education is to a large extent education for uncertainty. He told students:

> A distressing feature in the life which you are about to enter, a feature which will press hardly upon the finer spirits among you and ruffle their equanimity, is the uncertainty which pertains not alone to our science and art, but to the very hopes and fears which make us men. In seeking absolute truth we aim at the unattainable, and must be content with finding broken portions.[74]

Harking back to Hippocrates on another occasion, he noted:

> Listen to the appropriate comment of the Father of Medicine, who twenty-five centuries ago had not only grasped the fundamental conception of our art as one based on observation, but had laboured also through a long life to give to the profession which he loved the saving health of science—listen, I say, to the words of his famous aphorism: "*Experience is fallacious and judgment difficult!*" [75]

Like many but by no means most of his contemporaries, Osler was skeptical of the drug therapies of his day to the extent that he has been called a therapeutic nihilist. He was fond of quoting Oliver Wendell Holmes's famous saying that if all of the world's drugs were thrown into the oceans it would be good for humans and bad for fish. However, Osler did prescribe most of the available drugs that have since been shown to have a rational basis. He even experimented with acupuncture.[76] However, he adamantly opposed therapies that he thought were of little benefit. He was especially opposed to drug combinations: "The battle against poly-pharmacy, or the use of a large number of drugs (of the action of which we know little, yet we put them into bodies of the action of which we know less), has not been fought to a finish." [77] He strongly opposed misleading pharmaceutical advertising:

> Far too large a section of the treatment of disease is to-day control-led by the big manufacturing pharmacists, who have enslaved us in a plausible pseudo-science. The remedy is obvious: give our stu-dents a first-hand acquaintance with disease and give them a thor-ough practical knowledge of the great drugs, and we will send out independent, clear-headed, cautious practitioners who will do their own thinking and be no longer at the mercy of a meretricious literature which has sapped our independence.[78]

Among his favorite prescriptions was "time, in divided doses." [79] And he was not against the use of placebos, saying that one particular preparation "combines the three essentials [of a medi-cine]—color, taste, and harmlessness." [80]

In summary, Osler took a strong stand for intellectual honesty. It was probably no coincidence that he prefaced his textbook of medicine with a quotation from Plato's *Gorgias*: "And I said of medicine, that this is an art which considers the constitution of the patient, and has principles of action and reasons in each case." Gorgias was a Greek philosopher whose fame rests largely on a treatise entitled "On That Which Is Not, or On Nature," in which he went so far as to question whether anything exists at all.

BE BOTH TEACHER AND STUDENT

Osler saw nothing negative about the term "perpetual student." He said, "It goes without saying that no man can teach successfully who is not at the same time a student." [81] He accepted the invita-tion to join the faculty of the new medical school at Johns Hopkins because "a type of medical school was to be created new to this country in which teacher and student alike should be in the fighting line." [82] He treated students with mutual respect. At Johns Hopkins, this may have come about naturally enough because of uniquely stringent admission requirements that included a proficiency in French, German, biology, chemistry, and physics.[83] When the school opened, Osler is said to have remarked to his colleague William H. Welch, "Welch, it is lucky that we get in as professors; we never could enter as students." [84] The students were rewarded with what seems to have been a joyous experience. One student recalled that

> to those privileged to be his students in the early days of the medical school—a truly golden age to each and every one of the small, though ever-growing group, he preached, as he lived, a glorious philosophy of life, a joy in work, doing the day's tasks, "living for the day and for the day's work," with a wonderful belief in his fellow-men, never losing faith because some had failed him, giving without stint his best to everyone with no thought that some might prove unworthy of the trust. . . . To us who were his students in the early days of The Johns Hopkins Medical School, his memory is so vivid, so fresh, that it seems but as of yesterday when he worked and played in our midst.[85]

Another young man recalled that Osler

> pointed out problems, encouraged everyone in what he desired to do, and was more than liberal in his commendation of work done. His absolute generosity threw open his whole clinical material to the use of anyone who had a problem. He urged and assisted in the publication of the results, and saw to it that the young men got the whole credit of the work when often it should have gone to himself. Is it to be wondered at that such a chief has such devoted followers?[86]

Osler thus encouraged the students to join him as fellow learners, to write up their observations for medical journals, to attend medical meetings with him, and to feel in every way that they belonged to a vibrant, idealistic profession.[87] Yet while he treated students as fellow learners, Osler encouraged them to develop sound study habits:

> It is much simpler to buy books than to read them and easier to read them than to absorb their contents. Too many men slip early out of the habit of studious reading, and yet this is essential to a man if he is to get an education. To be worth anything it must be associated with concentration—with that mental application which means real effort.[88]

He also encouraged students to press on especially because of his conviction that true creativity occurs mainly before age 40 (see Chapters 3 and 7). It followed that teachers had much to gain by daily company with "younger, more receptive" minds:

> It is this loss of mental elasticity which makes men over forty so slow to receive new truths. Harvey complained in his day that few men above this critical age seemed able to accept the doctrine of the circulation of the blood, and in our own time it is interesting to note how the theory of the bacterial origin of certain diseases has had, as other truths, to grow to acceptance with the generation in which it was announced. The only safeguard in the teacher against this lamentable condition is to live . . . in company with the younger, more receptive and progressive minds.[89]

To encourage good reading habits and to promote exchange of ideas, Osler endorsed informal forums known as journal clubs. Although now commonplace, such clubs were not widespread in Osler's time. In Montreal and in Philadelphia, he started "foreign periodical clubs" to promote keeping up with the literature. At Johns Hopkins, he launched "The Journal Club," which met in the library "to enable all members of the staff to keep fully informed as to what is being accomplished by workers in every branch of medical science with the least expenditure of time."[90] It was perhaps in his effort to keep up with the medical literature that Osler showed most clearly his commitment to students of all ages. He was always distressed by the inability of many physicians to make time for reading. Visiting the Medical Library Association in Belfast in 1909, Osler made what Cushing called

> one of his characteristic addresses. . . . He emphasized the importance of reading as a part of post-graduate study. There had been men whose only book was nature, but these were the exceptions. The average non-reading doctor might play a good game of golf or of bridge, but professionally he was a lost soul. The driven and tired practitioner might plead that he could not find time to read. He could not unless he had formed the practice in less busy days; then the habit of reading, like any other habit, became his master. He should get away from the notion that it was necessary to read much. One or two journals and a few books every year were enough, if read properly. Journals should be kept and filed for reference, and all reading should be done with that mental concentration which made reading profitable. . . . He urged on the meeting the collection of

books on a definite system as the best of hobbies for the medical man.[91]

Lifelong learning was thus a recurrent theme of Osler's teaching. The original title of "The Student Life," one of his most popular addresses, was "The Student Aged 17 to 70." [92] In it he said:

> The hardest conviction to get into the mind of a beginner is that the education upon which he is engaged is not a college course, not a medical course, but a life course, for which the work of a few years under teachers is but a preparation. Whether you will falter and fail in the race or whether you will be faithful to the end depends on the training before the start, and on your staying powers, points upon which I need not enlarge. You can all become good students, a few may become great students, and now and again one of you will be found who does easily and well what others cannot do at all, or very badly, which is John Ferriar's excellent definition of a genius.[93]

This commitment to lifelong learning prompted Osler's practice of "quinquennial brain-dusting"—going abroad to clear his mind of routine and learn from colleagues in different places. He began this practice at 28 when he went to England to brush up on his knowledge. His biographer felt that his short sabbaticals "had no little influence in keeping him always in the front rank." [94] He stressed to teachers as well as students the importance of continual learning:

> Undoubtedly the student tries to learn too much, and we teachers try to teach him too much—neither, perhaps with great success. The existing evils result from neglect on the part of the teacher, student and examiner of the great fundamental principle laid down by Plato—that education is a life-long process, in which the student can only make a beginning during his college course. . . . We can only instil principles, put the student in the right path, give him methods, teach him how to study, and early to discern between essentials and non-essentials.[95]

But while Osler formed at an early age definite ideas about education, the real key to his success was personal interest. He urged his students on: "Take notes; publish; make yourself known." He asked about their progress.[96] He insisted that they be involved in meaningful clinical activities.[97] And he saw the educational process itself as a dynamic subject that deserved ongoing scrutiny and refinement.

REFINE THE METHODS

Osler's lasting contributions to medical education were in two areas. First, he improved the curriculum and popularized bedside clinical teaching. Second, he promoted research and thus enriched medicine's knowledge base. In both cases his contributions, while not unique, had major impacts on medicine.

Osler often receives credit for introducing bedside teaching for medical students, but he never made that claim. The practice dates at least to the seventeenth century, when Franciscus Sylvius began to teach students beside his 12 beds at a hospital in Leyden, Holland. Bedside teaching quickly gained such influential advocates as Hermann Boerhaave in Holland and Thomas Sydenham in England, became well-developed in Scotland, and as early as 1845 was being practiced at McGill, where Osler no doubt absorbed it.[98] In 1867 Holmes of Boston told Harvard students that the "most essential part of a student's instruction is obtained . . . not in the lecture-room, but at the bedside." [99] However, such bedside teaching was not widely available before Osler institutionalized the practice at Johns Hopkins. Returning there for a visit in 1914, he could say with pardonable pride that bedside teaching was "a method, initiated in Holland, developed in Edinburgh, matured in London, and long struggled for here [North America], but never attained until the Johns Hopkins Medical School was started." [100] Perhaps Osler's strongest statement on bedside teaching came in 1902 during an address at the New York Academy of Medicine. At most of the New York hospitals, students were barred from the wards and taught mainly in amphitheaters. It was on that occasion that Osler stated how his epitaph should read: "Here lies the man who admitted students to the wards." And he accurately predicted that "within the next quarter of a century the larger universities of this country will have their own hospitals in which the problems of nature known as disease will be studied as thoroughly as are those of Geology or Sanscrit." [101] Osler's emphasis on ward teaching applied mainly to fourth-year (senior) medical students. The third-year students spent most of their time in the outpatient clinic—a point that is now being reemphasized as the "Oslerian basis of education in the ambulatory setting." [102] Osler did not originate the practice of getting students directly involved with patients, but he used the method so successfully that others copied it and it became the norm.

But Osler's emphasis on teaching medical students was less on where to teach medicine than how to teach it. As he put it,

> The problem of all others which is perplexing the teacher to-day is not so much what to teach, but how to teach it, more especially how far and in what subjects the practical shall take the place of didactic teaching. . . . Slowly but surely practical methods are everywhere taking the place of theoretical teaching, but there will, I think, always be room in a school for the didactic lecture.[103]

He was passionately committed to curriculum reform and urged that

> the student needs more time for quiet study, fewer classes, fewer lectures, and, above all, the incubus of examinations should be lifted from his soul. To replace the Chinese by the Greek spirit would enable him to seek knowledge for itself, without a thought of the end, tested and taught day by day, the pupil and teacher working together on the same lines, only one a little ahead of the other. This is the ideal towards which we should move.[104]

Speaking to the Society of Internal Medicine in 1901, he emphasized what he called "the natural method" of teaching medicine:

> In the natural method of teaching the student begins with the patient, continues with the patient, and ends his studies with the patient, using books and lectures as tools, as means to an end. The student starts, in fact, as a practitioner, as an observer and repairer of disordered machines, with the structure and orderly functions of which he is perfectly familiar.[105]

As his career progressed, he had more control over his educational environment and could implement his methods more effectively.

Even more important than his methods was his personal touch. He did not flaunt his knowledge of medicine. At the bedside, he nearly always confined his remarks to what he had actually seen, heard, felt, and smelled. In this setting he seldom recited the medical literature or drifted off into theory. One student recalled that even in the preclinical years, "It was Sir William's custom to dash into various laboratories and often ask disconcerting anatomical questions of students who were dissecting or to look down the microscopes and inspect the slides of those studying pathology and bacteriology." [106] Such enthusiasm was naturally contagious.

Osler's promotion of medical science is less well known than his promotion of medical education, but it is equally important. As early as 1884, he said:

> It is one thing to know thoroughly and be able to teach well any given subject in a college, it is quite another thing to be able to take up that subject and by original work and investigation add to our stock of knowledge concerning it, or throw light upon the dark problems which may surround it. Many a man, pitchforked, so to speak, by local exigencies into a professional position has done the former well, but unless a man of extraordinary force he cannot break the invidious bar of defective training which effectually shuts him off from the latter and higher duties of his position.[107]

Experimentation was the essential basis for human progress: "The ancients thought as clearly as we do, had greater skills in the arts and architecture, but had never learned the use of the great instrument which has given man control over nature—experiment." [108] In an unpublished manuscript he took an even broader view of experimentation in its historic context:

> Philosophy, as Plato tells us, begins with wonder; and, staring open-eyed at the starry heavens on the plains of Mesopotamia, man took his first step in the careful observation of Nature, which carried him a long way in his career. But he was very slow to learn the second step—how to interrogate Nature—to search out her secrets, as Harvey puts it, by way of experiment. The Chaldeans who invented the gnomon, and predicted eclipses, made a good beginning. The Greeks did not get much beyond trained observation, though Pythagoras made one fundamental experiment when he determined the dependence of the pitch of sound on the length of the vibrating cord. . . . Man can do a great deal by observation and thinking, but with them alone he cannot unravel the mysteries of Nature. Had he been able, the Greeks would have done it; and could Plato and Aristotle have grasped the value of experiment in the progress of human knowledge the course of European history might have been very different.[109]

Osler himself seldom experimented but admired those who did. He liked to quote the advice John Hunter gave Edward Jenner, who devised an inoculation against smallpox: "Don't think, try!" [110] He especially admired such nineteenth-century clinicians as Laennec, who invented the stethoscope, and Louis, who introduced medical statistics. Of the former, he wrote that

> Laënnec really created clinical medicine as we know it to-day. The discovery of auscultation was only an incident, of vast moment it is true, in a systematic study of the correlation of symptoms with anatomical changes.[111]

And of the latter,

> Louis introduced what is known as the Numerical Method, a plan which we use every day, though the phrase is not now very often on our lips. The guiding motto of his life was "Ars medica tota in observationibus [the whole art of medicine is in observation]," in carefully observing facts, carefully collating them, carefully analysing them.[112]

He also admired Claude Bernard, the great French experimentalist who said: "When entering a laboratory one should leave theories in the cloakroom." [113] And he admired the spirit of scientific medicine in the German universities:

> No secondary motives sway their minds, no cry reaches them in the recesses of their laboratories, "of what practical utility is your work?" but, unhampered by social or theological prejudices, they have been able to cherish "the truth which has never been deceived—that complete truth which carries with it the antidote against the bane and danger which follow in the train of half-knowledge." [114]

With these models in mind, Osler did an enormous amount to nurture scientific medicine in the United States.

Osler underscored the value of the scientific method even for those who do not make science their careers:

> Unless scientific, a man gets no true perspective as he looks out on the world in action. . . . By scientific I do not mean the acquisition of the bare facts of science, but an understanding of its methods, a realisation of its meaning and an inoculation with its spirit. It is an attitude of mind, a sort of reflex, which at once on the presentation of a problem makes a man burn until its solution is accomplished, until he knows the status of the question among the investigators of the world.[115]

And again:

> To the physician particularly a scientific discipline is an incalculable gift, which leavens his whole life, giving exactness to his whole life, giving exactness to habits of thought and tempering the mind with that judicious faculty of distrust which can alone, amid the uncertainties of practice, make him wise unto salvation. For perdition inevitably awaits the mind of the practitioner who has never had the full inoculation with the leaven, who has never grasped clearly the relations of science to his art, and who knows nothing, and perhaps cares less, for the limitations of either.[116]

Osler gave much thought to the role of science in clinical medicine. On the one hand, he encouraged young physicians to be research-oriented: "With a system of fellowships and research scholarships a university may have a body of able young men, who on the outposts of knowledge are exploring, surveying, defining and correcting." [117] On the other hand, he knew that it would be difficult for young persons who had been trained primarily as clinicians to compete with basic scientists. In this respect, he was in some ways ahead of his time:

> One thing is certain; we clinicians must go to the physiologists, the pathologists and the chemists—they no longer come to us. To our irreparable loss these sciences have become so complicated and demand such life-long devotion that no longer do physiologists . . . become surgeons, chemists [become] clinicians, and saddest of all, the chair of pathology is no longer a stepping stone to the chair of medicine. The new conditions must be met if progress is to be maintained.[118]

Although Osler may have been ambivalent about the ability of a clinical teacher to undertake original investigation, he encouraged this activity especially by spreading goodwill and cooperation through organizations. Among the last things he did before leaving the United States was to help start the Inter-Urban Clinical Club, which enabled physician-investigators from various cities in the eastern United States to get together on a social and intellectual basis and share work in progress. The Inter-Urban Clinical Club became a model for similar ones throughout the country. An Oslerian tradition of useful cooperation infused the academic community, and the result was a golden age of medical education and research the likes of which the world had never known.

6

CARE

CAREFULLY

The Least Sentimental and the Most Helpful

Two images of Osler seem paradoxical. On the one hand he was the consummate caring and compassionate physician, "family doctor to the world," [1] a model of humanism, the embodiment of the Hippocratic ideal that "where there is love of man, there is also love of the art." Indeed, he quoted that ideal in his last major address, extolling the physician's

love of humanity associated with the love of his craft!—philanthropia and philotechnia—the joy of working joined in each one to a true love of his brother. Memorable sentence indeed! in which for the first time was coined the magic word *philanthropy*, and conveying the subtle suggestion that perhaps in this combination the longings of humanity may find their solution, and Wisdom—philosophia—at last be justified of her children. [2]

Yet on the other hand he was the self-controlled and emotionally restrained professional, Mr. Cool, a model of objectivity, the embodiment of *Aequanimitas*—his motto and the title of a famous address in which he urged young physicians to keep their composure. Can we reconcile these images? Some critics have said no. One, in an essay entitled "Against Aequanimitas," claimed that "the major voice that seems to emerge from all the serious, uplifting advice is the public tone of the academic snob." [3] Is Osler a useful role model? Was he the kind of doctor we want?

Osler seldom if ever pontificated about caring and compassion, perhaps because the subject was not one for serious debate when doctors could often offer little else. Things are different today. Doctors can do much more, yet socioeconomic forces at work to redefine medicine make caring an increasingly important subject. Such terms as managed care, capitated lives, product lines, cost-benefit ratios, economic credentialing, and risk sharing mandate close attention to what it is that doctors do and patients buy. [4] Are doctors strictly required only to render services within their realms of competence? Are they also obligated to be caring, concerned, and compassionate? If so, what do we mean by these terms and how can we measure them? Another issue is physician burnout. How should doctors care for themselves? Osler seems to have cared mainly with deeds rather than words, to have cared frequently rather than intensely, and to have cared for himself as well as others. Although his style may not be for everyone, he worked out a way to care effectively.

SHOW COMPASSION

Osler cared mainly through action, not words. His verbal displays of sympathy were nearly always short. Joseph Pratt's year-long diary of a Johns Hopkins clinic suggests Osler's preoccupation with the practical aspects of diagnosis and treatment. On one occasion, Osler and his students saw a man with angina pectoris (chest pain due to coronary artery disease) who chewed half a pound of tobacco a week. Two months later, he was still chewing tobacco and having chest pain. Osler told the student to "write him that he is a fool." After another two months the patient had stopped using tobacco and was pain-free. [5] An Oxford medical student wrote his mother that Osler had said "that *his rule had been to like and sympathize with everyone*. That's his creed, I think. He is the least sentimental and the most helpful man I've ever seen—the most lovable." [6]

How did Osler do it? Let us consider three examples.

At age 26, as a young professor at McGill, Osler often took his meals at the Metropolitan Club. There he met and sometimes joined at dinner a young Englishman who was in Montreal on business. One evening the guest appeared ill. Osler diagnosed smallpox and arranged a consultation with Dr. Palmer Howard. The young man was admitted to a special hospital for smallpox and died three days later. Osler ascertained the address of the young man's father and wrote a factual account of the course of events. He told how the young man had spoken "of his home, & his mother, and asked me to read the 43rd Chapter of Isaiah, which she had marked in his Bible." He told how death had come "without a groan or struggle" and how, as "the son of a clergyman & knowing well what it is to be a 'stranger in a strange land,' I performed the last office of Christian friendship I could, & read the Commendatory Prayer at his departure." Thirty years later, in England, Osler met a woman who recounted that her younger brother had died in Montreal, where he had "been cared for during a fatal illness by a doctor named Osler, who had sent a sympathetic letter that had been the greatest solace to her parents." Osler visited the mother and gave her a photograph of her son's grave that he had arranged to have taken.[7]

The second example concerns the way Osler carried out his duties at the almshouse at Ewelme, an ancient and picturesque village between Oxford and London. In 1437 the Duke of Suffolk and his wife Alice (who happened to be Chaucer's granddaughter) established the almshouse to provide security to 13 elderly men chosen from among the poor of that area. In 1546 King Henry VIII established the position of Regius Professor of Medicine at Oxford at a stipend of 40 pounds a year, and in 1617 King James I began what became a custom of making the regius professor also the Master of Ewelme to augment the regius professor's meager salary. Before Osler, most regius professors regarded the position of Master of Ewelme as little more than a sinecure. When Osler learned of the position, he resolved to take it seriously. He went regularly, got to know the old men, required them to fulfill their historic obligation to pray for their benefactress, brought friends and guests over to visit, organized picnics, and occasionally spent the night there. The morale at Ewelme and the general outlook of the elderly pensioners rose dramatically.[8]

The third example occurred on a day when Osler, on his way to an Oxford graduation ceremony and dressed in academic gown, was asked to see a small boy with severe whooping cough complicated by bronchitis. The child would not eat. The nurses and his parents tried to feed him without success. Osler did not have much time but acted as though he had plenty. He examined the child briefly and then sat down at the bedside. He carefully peeled a peach, coated it with sugar, cut it into small pieces, and offered them to the child one at a time, telling the boy that it was a special fruit and that he would find it good. Hurrying off to the ceremony, he gave the boy's father a bleak prognosis: "I'm sorry Ernest but I don't think I shall see the boy again, there's very little chance when they're bad as that." Osler visited the child daily for 40 days. Because the boy had seen him as a magical figure in his academic regalia, Osler brought his robe and put it on outside the room before each visit. The child began to improve a few days after the first visit and made a full recovery.[9]

Osler's emotional reactions to these and similar episodes are largely unknown. He did not make "I feel . . ." statements about his caring and concern. Instead he went the extra mile when it might make a difference. Nothing obligated him to write the young Englishman's father, nor did he have reason to think that he would ever see the young man's family. Nothing obligated him to befriend the old men at Ewelme, nor did they have anything to give except their appreciation. Nothing obligated him to make daily visits to the child with whooping cough, much less go to the trouble to bring his academic gown. But in each instance he went out of his way to do something that was both kind and substantial. It was through these and countless similar acts that Osler gained his reputation as the quintessential humanitarian, the paradigm of the caring doctor. As an adulatory medical student wrote of Osler's clinics, "I came away impressed by the greatness of Dr. Osler, his sincerity, his simplicity, his love for mankind and his desire to be of help to others." [10]

Although he seldom if ever waxed eloquent about "compassion," Osler recognized the importance of sympathy and charity in medicine. In the introduction to his history of medicine, he declared:

> Medicine arose out of the primal sympathy of man with man; out of the desire to help those in sorrow, need and sickness.

> In the primal sympathy
> Which having been must ever be;
> In the soothing thoughts that spring
> Out of human suffering.

> The instinct of self-preservation, the longing to relieve a loved one, and above all, the maternal passion—for such it is—gradually softened the hard race of man—*tum genus humanum primum mollescere cœpit* [Then the human race first began to grow soft].[11]

He held charity to be essential to the practice of medicine:

> As the practice of medicine is not a business and can never be one, the education of the heart—the moral side of the man—must keep pace with the education of the head. Our fellow creatures cannot be dealt with as man deals in corn and coal; "the human heart by which we live" must control our professional relations.[12]

Indeed, Osler held that helping others was the single most distinctive aspect of medicine. Addressing the Canadian Medical Association in 1902, he remarked that

> the profession of medicine is distinguished from all others by its *singular beneficence*. It alone does the work of charity in a Jovian and God-like way, dispensing with free hand truly Promethean gifts. There are those who listen to me who have seen three of the most benign endowments granted to the race since the great Titan stole fire from the heavens. Search the scriptures of human achievement and you cannot find any to equal in beneficence the introduction of Anæsthesia, Sanitation, with all that it includes, and Asepsis—a short half century's contribution towards the practical solution of the problems of human suffering, regarded as eternal and insoluble.[13]

One contemporary said that Osler's unspoken motto seemed to have been "Do the kind thing, and do it first." [14]

How did Osler reconcile the need to be compassionate with the need to be calm and objective—the message of his famous address "Aequanimitas"? The obvious answer was that there must be a balance: "The physician needs a clear head and a kind heart; his work is arduous and complex, requiring the exercise of the very highest faculties of the mind, while constantly appealing to the emotions and finer feelings." [15] In 1897 Osler told an audience of nurses:

> To measure finely and nicely your sympathy in these cases is a very delicate operation. The individual temperament controls the situation, and the more mobile of you will have a hard lesson to learn in subduing your emotions. It is essential, however, and never let your outward action demonstrate the native act and figure of your heart. You are lost irrevocably, should you so far give the reins to your feelings as to "ope the sacred source of sympathetic tears." Do enter upon your duties with a becoming sense of your frailties.

Yet he reminded the nurses of their unique opportunity to be charitable:

> In Institutions the corroding effect of routine can be withstood only by maintaining high ideals of work; but these become the sounding brass and tinkling cymbals without corresponding sound practice. In some of us the ceaseless panorama of suffering tends to dull that fine edge of sympathy with which we started. A great corporation cannot have a very fervent charity; the very conditions of its existence limit the exercise. Against this benumbing influence, we physicians and nurses, the immediate agents of the Trust, have but one enduring corrective—the practice towards patients of the Golden Rule of Humanity as announced by Confucius: "What you do not like when done to yourself, do not do to others,"—so familiar to us in its positive form as the great Christian counsel of perfection, in which alone are embraced both the law and the prophets.

He assured them: "There is no higher mission in this life than nursing God's poor." [16] It was similarly recalled that he told medical students, "Never forget the rights of patients." [17]

Three aspects of Osler's humanism deserve further comment. First, he taught that involvement in the lives of everyday people bestows an enormous blessing in return:

> Nothing will sustain you more potently than the power to recognize in your humdrum routine, as perhaps it may be thought, the true poetry of life—the poetry of the commonplace, of the ordinary man,

of the plain, toil-worn woman, with their loves and their joys, their sorrows and their griefs.[18]

Speaking informally to students at Oxford, he told them, "In my behavior to my patients I make no difference whatever between the high and the low, between a duchess and a cook." [19]

Second, he recognized the value of psychological factors including faith (see also Chapter 8). In the seventh edition of his textbook of medicine, he wrote:

> In all ages, and in all lands, the prayer of faith, to use the words of St. James, has healed the sick; and we must remember that amid the Æsculapian cult, the most elaborate and beautiful system of faith-healing the world has seen, scientific medicine took its rise. As a profession, consciously or unconsciously, more often the latter, *faith* has been one of our most valuable assets, and Galen expressed a great truth when he said, "He cures most successfully in whom the people have the greatest confidence." [20]

Many persons vouched for his effectiveness at psychotherapy.[21] A student recalled him "with a smile or an epigram for every doctor and nurse who passed, a kindly word, and his ever-stimulating psychotherapy—encouragement, optimism, hope—to every patient he saw." [22] A colleague remembered that "when he had gone there was a feeling that everything was all right. The visit was nearly always marked by some cheering saying or amusing quip." [23] Still another wrote that Osler's patients usually "carried away with them some felicitous phrase that had a greater healing effect than the written prescription." [24] Attributed to Osler by oral tradition is the exhortation "Never leave the bedside without a word of encouragement."

Finally, he was sincere and it showed. Patients trusted him. As an Oxford physician put it,

> No one with the least feeling for the mind of his fellows could be in Osler's presence for two minutes without feeling that here was a man to whom a man could lay bare his mind, a man whom one could trust absolutely. While such an impression can easily be conveyed by a manner of sincerity, Osler's sincerity was no mere cultivated manner; his sincerity was so pure as to be effortless.[25]

Cushing noted that Osler had an unusual ability to sympathize with and understand people.[26] Osler's cousin Jennette observed:

> Of self-conceit or boastfulness he had not a trace; he thought for others and seemed to forget himself. The servants would gladly do anything possible for him; he had the happy knack of friendliness to rich and poor, young and old, learned and ignorant; and what he was in character as a boy and young man he continued to be throughout his life: an out-giving, expressing nature, sympathetic and true.[27]

Although Osler sought to be efficient on his ward rounds, avoiding the ever-present danger of getting bogged down in conversation to the detriment of getting his work done, he was nevertheless sensitive to those around him. And if he did not lecture about compassion, he extolled the value of service to others. Thus he closed his review of Burton's *Anatomy of Melancholy* with the recognition that serving others repays us manyfold and is a good way to fight depression:

> We can best oppose any tendency to melancholy by an active life of unselfish devotion to others; and with the advice with which Burton ends the book, I will close:
>
> > 'Give not way to solitariness and idleness . . .
> >
> > Sperate miseri;
> > Cavete fœlices.'
> >
> > If unhappy, have hope;
> > If happy, be cautious.[28]

And on this point one of Osler's aphorisms seems especially unforgettable: "Care more particularly for the individual patient than for the special features of the disease." [29]

MAINTAIN EQUANIMITY

As Osler prepared to leave Philadelphia for Baltimore in 1889, he was asked to give the valedictory address to the graduating medical students at the University of Pennsylvania. The result was one of his shortest but most famous addresses, "Aequanimitas." He said at the outset that he was going to focus on but two of many elements that the graduates would find necessary:

> I could have the heart to spare you, poor, careworn, survivors of a hard struggle, so "lean and pale and leaden-eyed with study;" and my tender mercy constrains me to consider but two of the score of elements which may make or mar your lives—which may contribute to your success, or help you in the days of failure.

The first of these elements was imperturbability and the second was *aequanimitas*.

He began the lecture by talking about imperturbability, which he considered a physical attribute:

> In the first place, in the physician or surgeon no quality takes rank with imperturbability, and I propose for a few minutes to direct your attention to this essential bodily virtue. . . . Imperturbability means coolness and presence of mind under all circumstances, calmness amid storm, clearness of judgment in moments of grave peril, immobility, impassiveness, or, to use an old and expressive word, *phlegm*. It is the quality which is most appreciated by the laity though often misunderstood by them; and the physician who has the misfortune to be without it, who betrays indecision and worry, and who knows that he is flustered and flurried in ordinary emergencies, loses rapidly the confidence of his patients.

He suggested that some people are naturally imperturbable while others can never attain this attribute, but that most people could improve with practice:

> In full development, as we see it in some of our older colleagues, it has the nature of a divine gift, a blessing to the possessor, a comfort to all who come in contact with him. . . . As imperturbability is largely a bodily endowment, I regret to say that there are those amongst you, who, owing to congenital defects, may never be able to acquire it. Education, however, will do much; and with experience the majority of you may expect to attain a fair measure.

Osler suggested two ways for cultivating this trait, the first of which was to make a conscious effort to control one's display of emotions:

> The first essential is to have your nerves well in hand. Even under the most serious circumstances, the physician or surgeon who allows "his outward action to demonstrate the native act and figure

of his heart in complement extern," who shows in his face the slightest alteration, expressive of anxiety or fear, has not his medullary centres under the highest control, and is liable to disaster at any moment. I have spoken of this to you on many occasions, and have urged you to educate your nerve centres so that not the slightest dilator or contractor influence shall pass to the vessels of your face under any professional trial. Far be it from me to urge you, ere Time has carved with his hours those fair brows, to quench on all occasions the blushes of ingenuous shame, but in dealing with your patients emergencies demanding these should certainly not arise, and at other times an inscrutable face may prove a fortune.

The second measure was to know, through knowledge and experience, precisely what to do:

In a true and perfect form, imperturbability is indissolubly associated with wide experience and an intimate knowledge of the varied aspects of disease. With such advantages he is so equipped that no eventuality can disturb the mental equilibrium of the physician; the possibilities are always manifest, and the course of action is clear.

He went on to acknowledge that such lack of emotion might be seen by outsiders as hard-heartedness:

From its very nature this precious quality is liable to be misinterpreted, and the general accusation of hardness, so often brought against the profession, has here its foundation. Now a certain measure of insensibility is not only an advantage, but a positive necessity in the exercise of a calm judgment, in carrying out delicate operations. Keen sensibility is doubtless a virtue of high order, when it does not interfere with steadiness of hand or coolness of nerve; but for the practitioner in his working-day world, a callousness which thinks only of the good to be effected, and goes ahead regardless of smaller considerations, is the preferable quality.

Concluding, he urged:

Cultivate, then, gentlemen such a judicious measure of obtuseness as will enable you to meet the exigencies of practice with firmness and courage, without, at the same time, hardening "the human heart by which we live."

Thus Osler did not deny the value of compassion (or "keen sensibility"). He merely said that losing control of one's emotions or "nerves" can cloud accurate diagnosis and sound judgment.

Osler introduced *aequanimitas* as the mental counterpart to the physical attribute of imperturbability:

> In the second place, there is a mental equivalent to this bodily endowment, which is as important in our pilgrimage as imperturbability. Let me recall to your minds an incident related of that best of men and wisest of rulers, Antoninus Pius, who, as he lay dying, in his home at Lorium in Etruria, summed up the philosophy of life in the watchword, *Aequanimitas*. As for him, about to pass *flammantia moenia mundi* (the flaming ramparts of the world), so for you, fresh from Clotho's spindle [the web of fate], a calm equanimity is the desirable attitude. How difficult to attain, yet how necessary, in success as in failure! Natural temperament has much to do with its development, but a clear knowledge of our relation to our fellow-creatures and to the work of life is also indispensable.

Aequanimitas is thus mental calmness that "is chiefly exercised in enabling us to bear with composure the misfortunes of our neighbours." [30] Osler was much admired for his ability to stay calm in trying circumstances, such as meetings in which people were losing their tempers. Those who knew him well suspected that, like the rest of us, he had to work at it. Thomas McCrae vouched that "many who came in contact with him never realized how much anxiety he often felt, but rarely displayed over patients. This was particularly true if it was a case in which a diagnosis had not been made and in which, therefore, the best treatment was a question of doubt." [31] Osler admired the quality of calmness in others. In his eulogy to Alfred Stillé he suggested that aequanimitas improves with advancing years, noting that Stillé "had that delightful equanimity and serenity of mind which is one of the most blessed accompaniments of old age." [32] Osler himself was not immune to occasional displays of anxiety, disappointment, frustration, and anger.[33] Imperturbability and aequanimitas, like other virtues, should be viewed as ideals to which we aspire knowing that we will sometimes fall short. Osler made this clear when he concluded his address: "Gentlemen,—Farewell, and take with you into the struggle the watchword of the good old Roman—*Aequanimitas*." [34]

TOUCH FREQUENTLY

Much of Osler's influence with patients, pupils, and peers can be attributed to those magical qualities that, for want of a better word, we summarize as charisma. As one person put it, he "had an extraordinary power of attracting men to him; though exactly why every one loved him so much is . . . difficult to say." Closer analysis reveals that he reinforced his charisma by two practices that anyone can emulate. First, he practiced touching the lives of others on a frequent but not intense basis. Second, he often played with children and related to them in a childlike fashion.

Marcia Grad, in her book *Charisma: How to Get "That Special Magic,"* lists characteristics that charismatic persons have "in extraordinary amounts—high energy, sustained vitality, courage, composure (especially when under stress), strong sense of self, clear direction and movement toward one's goal or goals, and determination to succeed." [35] Other qualities of charismatic persons include (1) showing interest in others on a frequent and regular basis, satisfying their needs, and shining the spotlight on them; (2) putting others at ease, helping them to feel comfortable, without boasting or consciously trying to impress them; (3) projecting optimism and joy of living; (4) maintaining good body language and eye contact; (5) listening well; and (6) self-acceptance. Grad concludes that "we must work to develop the deep, sensitive, compassionate parts of ourselves, to routinely treat others gently and affectionately, to be aware of their motivations, and to be responsive to their needs." [36] If we wish to make a difference in others' lives by being special to them, we must find our own distinctive ways to reach their hearts.

Osler seldom indulged in long, soul-searching conversations. His policy was to affirm people in small but frequent increments by noticing, complimenting, encouraging, or simply exchanging information. Thus Cushing observed that in Baltimore, "Osler, debonair, in a grey frock-coat, top hat, and the inevitable nosegay in his buttonhole, passed no familiar spot without a visit and the leaving of a touching or humorous recollection in some one's mind." [37] These practices—contacting people regularly rather than intensely, praising them often rather than lavishly—are precisely those taught by today's experts on personnel management. Another time-efficient yet endearing habit of Osler's was his omission of the stereotyped "How have you been?" When he met someone whom he had not seen for a long time, he would jump right back into the relationship where it had left off, immediately expressing interest in the other person's activities.[38] Formalities, he seemed to say, were unimportant.

He also kept up with others by writing to an extent reminiscent of what Plutarch had to say about Alexander the Great: "It is in fact astonishing that he could find time to write so many letters to his friends." [39] Here too Osler favored frequency over intensity. One colleague observed that "he would in a few words convey his meaning and did not give way to sentiment. He was, in some respects, rather like Gladstone in that he communicated his wishes or his intentions by means of postcard." [40] Osler kept a supply of prestamped postcards handy at all times and dashed off brief notes as the spirit moved him, leaving the task of dating these messages to the post office. In this way he reminded friends and colleagues that they mattered without imposing an obligation to reciprocate his correspondence. Hundreds of Osler's postcards and short letters exist, and several collections have been published including Osler's extended correspondence with Charles N. B. Camac, a former pupil. While Camac typically wrote to "My Dear Dr. Osler," Osler's salutations were usually just "Dear Camac" and the letters almost invariably terse.[41] For example:

> *Dear Camac*: Your note of the 30th with the welcome news I found this p.m. on my return from Michigan. Many congratulations! Love to Mother & Child.
> *Yours ever, W. Osler*

And:

> *Dear Camac*: As I telegraphed you I could see Col. Weir with you about 4 p.m. I get to 232nd St. at 3:15. Send me word to the Club where to join you. I cannot stop with you [for] dinner as I have an engagement.
> *Sincerely yours, Wm. Osler*

When Osler saw an article or other accomplishment by a colleague or former pupil, he would often dash off a postcard with a short compliment or "golden brick." He knew that a sure way to feel good about oneself is to help others feel good about themselves.

Like many and perhaps most charismatic people, Osler honed his ability to reach the true selves of other people by spending time with children. Children tended to see him as one of them, and he in turn sometimes preferred their company over that of adults.[42] One of his favorite games on entering a house was to quietly hide the children's cat and then instigate a high-spirited search for the sequestered animal "until it was triumphantly recovered with shrieks and war whoops." [43] He loved to enthrall young audiences with tall tales drawn from his own fertile imagination. In Baltimore, he once arrived at a home during a rainstorm and told the children that the flooding had been so severe around Mount Vernon Place that he had escaped drowning only by wrapping his arms around the Washington Monument. At Oxford, a distinguished visitor who had not previously met Osler arrived at Osler's home and found the regius professor playing make-believe on the floor with a child. At one of the picnics at Ewelme, a mother frantically searched for her ten-year-old daughter only to find her carrying a new doll and walking hand-in-hand with a new friend whom she called "William."[44] He also wrote children letters. Thus he wrote an eight-year-old girl: "The Secretary of the High Cockolorum Lord Chancellor presents his compliments to Miss Muriel Brock & begs to inform her that the Lord Chancellor himself is at present engaged upon a handy manual dealing with the whole subject of table-manners for children." The letter was signed "Obadiah Tweedledum." [45] Another little girl, Susan Revere Baker, left her favorite shopworn doll, Rosalie, in Osler's care for a while. Osler diligently wrote Susan about Rosalie's progress.[46] Rosalie's "mother" later noted: "He would give up an important engagement, to have five o'clock supper with a little girl and her dolls, and no little girl could ever forget the joy of his presence, for he entered into the make-believe so genuinely." [47] And he maintained an interest in the children after they had grown up. He kept up a long correspondence with Marjorie Howard, the young daughter of a colleague, and when she had grown into a young woman flattered her with letters such as the following:

> Light of my later Life—adorable superba Absent from thee my heart languishes and I feel so desolated that neither my work nor play has any joy in it. With you and in your presence the smallest trifles of life are full of abiding happiness. That day you remember when I

had a bad oyster at dinner—your sympathetic glance alone gave me the courage to swallow it.[48]

"Charisma" comes from the Greek *kharisma*, meaning "divine favor." Osler augmented whatever natural charisma he may have had with a set of practices that are within anyone's reach, and in so doing, showed others that he cared about them in a way that was regular, ongoing, entertaining, and meaningful.

CARE FOR YOURSELF

Osler once wrote, "In no relationship is the physician more often derelict than in his duty to himself." [49] He was no doubt familiar with the advice of his mentor, Sir Thomas Browne, that "charity begins at home"—namely, with ourselves:

> 'Tis the general complaint of these times, and perhaps of those past, that charity grows cold; which I perceive most verified in those which most do manifest the fires and flames of zeal; for it is a virtue that best agrees with coldest natures, and such as are complexioned for humility: But how shall we expect charity towards others, when we are uncharitable to ourselves? Charity begins at home, is the voice of the world, yet is every man his own greatest enemy, and as it were, his own executioner.[50]

Indeed, Browne considered it fortunate that we die but once:

> Men that look no further than their outsides think health an appurtenance unto life, and quarrel with their constitutions for being sick; but I that have examined the parts of man, and know upon what tender filaments that Fabric hangs, do wonder that we are not always so; and considering the thousand doors that lead to death do thank my God that we can die but once.[51]

As William Osler's medical practice grew in his fifth decade, he became increasingly concerned about his own health and specifically about the possibility of coronary heart disease. In 1897 he wrote a monograph on angina pectoris and observed how common the disease was among doctors. He recognized that stress is a factor in its pathogenesis:

> In the worry and strain of modern life arterial degeneration is not only very common, but develops often at a relatively early age. For

this I believe that the high pressure at which men live, and the habits of working the machine to its maximum capacity, are responsible, rather than excesses in eating or drinking. . . . Angeio-sclerosis, creeping on slowly but surely, "with no pace perceived," is the Nemesis through which Nature exacts retributive justice for the transgression of her laws—coming to one as an apoplexy, to another as an early Bright's disease, to a third as an aneurysm, and to a fourth as angina pectoris, too often slitting "the thin spun life" in the fifth decade, at the very time when success seems assured.[52]

By that time, Osler's own success seemed indeed assured—but at such price! His reputation as the ultimate diagnostic authority drew patients from all over the Western Hemisphere. In 1901 he analyzed the extent of his outside work:

My professional work increased very much this year. I have analysed it as a matter of interest. There were 780 new patients (exclusive of private patients at the Hospital) of whom 378 came from outside the city—Md. 44; Washington city 59; Va. 57; W. Va. 21; Pa. 39; N.Y. City 22; N.Y. State 8; Ala. 15; Ohio 12; Ga. 7; Mo. 5; Ill. 7; Ind. 1; Del. 2; N.C. 20; S.C. 5; Mich. 4; Col. 2; Mont. 1; Fla. 2; Tex. 2; Cal. 2; Miss. 2; Utah 3; Wis. 2; Wash. 2; N.J. 4; La. 4; R.I. 2; Minn. 3; Mass. 4; Ky. 2; Quebec 5; Ont[ario] 9; N[ova]S[cotia] 1; Mex[ico] 2; W[est] I[ndies] 1—representing 31 states.[53]

In addition, he was out of town for professional reasons 33 times that year, and although most of the trips were to Washington, where he consulted at the White House, he went south to Florida and to Thomasville, Georgia, to see patients. He made more than $40,000 from seeing patients, quite a large sum at the time and tax-free, but the price was high. By 1903 he complained privately, "It becomes more and more difficult to meet outside demands." [54]

    It got worse. Then as now, many patients seeking diagnosis were the worried well whose symptoms defy organic explanation. Osler was usually effective at dealing with such people, but it took a great deal out of him. He had always opposed seeing patients quickly and making snap diagnoses. It was difficult to see so many patients and do the other things that he enjoyed, such as teaching, writing, editing, book collecting, being involved in public health issues of the day, serving through medical societies, and spending time with his friends. Yet he found it hard to say no especially to other physicians, who increasingly asked him to treat them and their families. He complained to a colleague: "I am living a 'life of the hunted' at present. Infernal nuisance & yet it seems very difficult to limit one's legitimate work." [55]

The solution was a less stressful job. In 1904 he was asked if he would consider the position of Regius Professor at Oxford, a prestigious appointment with light duties since Oxford had no medical school or university hospital. Osler wrote in his diary that such an appointment would "offer the chance of escape from an ever increasing pressure of work." He saw little chance of such escape in Baltimore. As he wrote later, "In spite of the most careful regulation of my time and health I was often utterly 'used up' at the end of the week, and the question was how long could I hold out at the high pressure." Still he equivocated. He told Sir John Burdon Sanderson, his former teacher who had just given up the position of Regius Professor, that he was deeply indebted to the medical profession in North America, "which had done so much for me." About July 31, 1904, however, he received a letter formally offering the position. It was then that Mrs. Osler, also concerned about his health, put her foot down: "Better to go in a steamer than go in a pine-box." [56] Taking her advice, Osler wrote in his diary:

> After an exchange of cables with Mrs. Osler I accepted. All along she was in favor of the change, feeling the pace of my present life could have but one ending—a serious breakdown. I arranged to spend the session in Baltimore. There was a perfect chorus of lamentations, lay and medical. In England the news of the appointment was very well received, tho all my friends wondered not a little that I should give up such a splendid clinical position for a comparative sinecure. Financially, of course, it meant a tremendous sacrifice, lopping off at least three fourths of my income, but with my book and what I had saved with the salary—which I knew was small, but about which I had not asked—and Mrs. Osler's private income—about $5000—I felt sure that we could live quietly and happily.[57]

With the decision to reduce the stress in his life, Osler had managed to heed his own advice. In 1903, at the height of his popularity as a clinician, he had told physicians in New Haven, Connecticut:

> Greater sympathy must be felt for a man who has started all right and has worked hard . . . but as the rolling years have brought

ever-increasing demands on his time, the evening hours find him worn and yet not able to rest. . . . Of all men in the profession the forty-visit-a-day man is the most to be pitied. Not always an automaton, he may sometimes by economy of words and extraordinary energy do his work well . . . [but] too often he is lost beyond all recall, and, like Ephraim joined to his idols, we may leave him alone. Many good men are ruined by success in practice.[58]

Yet he underscored personal responsibility for health whatever the external demands might be. By age 60 Osler may have been reflecting on his own case when he reflected on the prognosis of coronary heart disease:

Much depends on the patient himself—on the life he has led—the life he is willing to lead. The ordinary high-pressure business or professional man may find relief, or even cure, in the simple process of slowing the engines, reducing the speed from the 25 knots an hour of a *Lusitania* to the 10 knots of a "black Bilboa tramp." The difficulty is to induce a man of this type to lessen "the race, an' rack, an' strain." As William Pepper used to say: "Give me the life of a hare rather than the existence of a tortoise." Not even the terrible outbursts of pain may suffice to check men of this stamp. . . . We doctors are notorious sinners in this respect, but it is so hard to lessen work when in full swing, so much harder than to give it up altogether, and how few of us at 50 or 55 are able to do this![59]

And still later, he wrote:

I had thirty-one years of uninterrupted hard work. William Pepper, my predecessor in Philadelphia, died of angina at 55; John Musser, my successor, of the same disease at 53! After listening to my story you may wonder how it was possible to leave a place [Johns Hopkins] so gratifying to the ambitions of any clinical teacher: I had had a good innings and was glad to get away without a serious breakdown.[60]

Although he urged self-responsibility for health, he recognized that for many physicians, especially those in primary care practice, this can be a difficult matter:

Few men live lives of more devoted self-sacrifice than the family physician, but he may become so completely absorbed in work that leisure is unknown; he has scarce time to eat or to sleep, and, as Dr. Drummond remarks in one of his poems, "He's the only man, I know me, don't get no holiday." There is danger in this treadmill life lest he lose more than health and time and rest—his intellectual independence.[61]

This advice still rings true. Thus a recent medical school commencement speaker put it, "Keep your minds open, your hearts full, and your ears attuned to the calling. And, for goodness' sake, physicians, take care of yourselves!" [62]

KEEP A SENSE OF HUMOR

Medicine can be stressful for many reasons, especially the anxiety of uncertainty, the sorrows of dealing with the sick, and—perhaps more than anything else—the excruciating time pressures.[63] High among Osler's defense mechanisms against stress was an exceptional sense of humor (see also Chapter 4).[64] He was usually playful, full of fun, and capable of mirth at a moment's notice. Yet as one observer put it, "Never a man masked, so successfully, earnestness of purpose and a real love of his fellowmen with a glimmering veil of humour. He was most in earnest when he was most in fun." [65] Osler himself wrote, "Like song that sweetens toil, laughter brightens the road of life, and to be born with a sense of the comic is a precious heritage." [66] And as he told North American medical students during a 1905 farewell address, he held that doctors should be cheerful, able to laugh, and sensitive to the comic as well as the tragic side of life:

> The comedy, too, of life will be spread before you, and nobody laughs more often than the doctor at the pranks Puck [a mischievous sprite in fictional literature, such as Shakespeare's *Midsummer Night's Dream*] plays upon the Titanias and Bottoms among his patients. The humorous side is really almost as frequently turned towards him as the tragic. Lift up one hand to heaven and thank your stars if they have given you the proper sense to enable you to appreciate the inconceivably droll situations in which we catch our fellow creatures. Unhappily, this is one of the free gifts of the gods, unevenly distributed, not bestowed on all, or on all in equal portions. In undue measure it is not without risk, and in any case in

the doctor it is better appreciated by the eye than expressed on the tongue. Hilarity and good humour, a breezy cheerfulness, a nature "sloping toward the southern side," as Lowell has it, help enormously both in the study and in the practice of medicine. To many of a sombre and sour disposition it is hard to maintain good spirits amid the trials and tribulations of the day, and yet it is an unpardonable mistake to go about among patients with a long face.[67]

His humor was part and parcel of his caring.

Osler was not a teller of jokes or a maker of puns. One of his trademarks was the practical joke, a form of humor more typical of the Victorian era into which he was born than of our own. His boyhood friend Ned Milburn recalled: "The spirit of fun was well marked in him—real fun that hurt nobody but sometimes caused a little annoyance to the victims of the joke." [68] He mastered early in life the ability to mislead with plausible but erroneous facts delivered over a deadpan expression. There was, for example, the time that another man came to visit his father and Willie whispered to both of them that "you'll have to speak loudly—he's nearly deaf." Watching them shout at each other brought him so much pleasure that he would repeat the prank as an adult. He also liked to send people on wild goose chases. Once he told a McGill graduate when he left Baltimore for Philadelphia to "drop in on my old friends Philip Syng Physick and Shippen and give them my love." The young man spent the better part of the day in Philadelphia looking for Physick and Shippen only to learn that they were long dead. There was the time when Osler was in Montreal for a medical meeting and went unannounced to a dinner one of his friends was having for a Boston pediatrician who seemed to Osler to be excessively preoccupied with precise infant formulas. He asked the pediatrician's wife if she had visited the new suburb of Caughnawauga, across the river from Montreal, which had beautiful parks, schools, theaters, and an unusually fine children's hospital that incorporated the latest methods. The couple looked in vain for the mythical suburb before they realized that they had been duped. They never forgave him.[69]

Another characteristic expression of Osler's humor was the tall tale that progresses from the plausible to the impossible in such a way that the line between truth and fiction becomes blurred. On one occasion, the Johns Hopkins pathologist William MacCallum asked Osler at a dinner in New York "the name of this delicious fish we are eating." Osler replied, "It is a scrod." MacCallum exclaimed, "Scrod! I never heard of it!" Osler proceeded to give MacCallum an outlandish explanation:

> You know what a capon is; scrod is codfish that has received the same treatment. The production of scrod has become a thriving industry along the New England coast. . . . The cod come up inlets from the sea in great numbers in the spring and are diverted into narrow, shallow troughs, from which they are removed by the nimble hands of trained workers, who quickly and skilfully castrate them. They are then placed in large vats or artificial pools of salt water. There, after a month or so, their flesh acquires a new and improved flavor. They are then shipped to market.

Enthralled, MacCallum exclaimed, "It is most remarkable, and all new to me." [70] It is not known whether MacCallum eventually learned that "scrod" is merely a culinary term for a young codfish that has been split and boned.

The full flowering of such expressions of Osler's humor were thinly disguised by the *nom de plume* Egerton Yorrick Davis. Indeed, Egerton Yorrick Davis or EYD served Osler as an alter ego and reminder not to take himself too seriously. Davis was allegedly an assistant surgeon in the United States Army who had been stationed among the Caughnawauga Indians, who drowned in the Lachine Rapids in 1884, and whose body was never recovered. In 1882 Davis surfaced in a manuscript submitted to the *Canada Medical and Surgical Journal* entitled "Professional Notes among the Indian Tribes about the Great Slave Lake, North West Territory" that soberly related some highly unusual (and fictitious) tribal rites pertaining to virility, infertility, and child delivery. Osler confessed the joke to the editor, and the manuscript was not published at the time. But Osler did not confess to a later case report submitted to the Philadelphia *Medical News* as a practical joke on a member of that journal's editorial board, one Theophilus Parvin. Parvin was a leading but rather pompous obstetrician who had written a stilted essay about "penis captivis"—the condition in which a couple is made literally inseparable by coitus. Reproducing this note in its entirely should dispel any idea that Osler was himself pompous:

> *Dear Sir*: The reading of an admirably written and instructive editorial in the Philadelphia MEDICAL NEWS for 24th November, on

forms of vaginismus, has reminded me of a case in point which bears out, in an extraordinary way, the statements contained therein. When in practice in Pentonville, I was sent for, about 11 p.m., by a gentleman whom, on my arriving at his house, I found in a state of great perturbation, and the story he told me was briefly as follows:

At bedtime, when going to the back kitchen to see if the house was shut up, a noise in the coachman's room attracted his attention, and, going in, he discovered to his horror that the man was in bed with one of the maids. She screamed, he struggled, and they rolled out of bed together and made frantic efforts to get apart, but without success. He was a big, burly man, over six feet, and she was a small woman, weighing not more than ninety pounds. She was moaning and screaming, and seemed in great agony, so that, after several fruitless attempts to get them apart, he sent for me. When I arrived I found the man standing up and supporting the woman in his arms, and it was quite evident that his penis was tightly locked in her vagina, and any attempt to dislodge it was accompanied by much pain on the part of both. It was, indeed, a case of "De cohesione in coitu." I applied water, and then ice, but ineffectually, and at last sent for chloroform, a few whiffs of which sent the woman to sleep, relaxed the spasm, and relieved the captive penis which was swollen, livid, and in a state of semi-erection, which did not go down for several hours, and for days the organ was extremely sore. The woman recovered rapidly, and seemed none the worse.

I am sorry that I did not examine if the sphincter ani was contracted, but I did not think of it. In this case there must have been also spasm of the muscle at the orifice, as well as higher up, for the penis seemed nipped low down, and this contraction, I think, kept the blood retained and the organ erect. As an instance of Jago's "beast with two backs," the picture was perfect. I have often wondered how it was, considering with what agility the man can, under certain circumstances, jump up, that Phineas, the son of Eleazer, was able to thrust his javelin through the man and the Midianitish woman (*vide* Exodus); but the occurrence of such cases as the above may offer a possible explanation.

Yours truly, Egerton Y. Davis, Ex. U.S. Army

This story contains all of the elements of good satire. Plausible facts replete with minor details blend almost imperceptibly with the outlandish, yet the ultimate aim is instructive. In this and similar satires, Osler followed the style of the French writer François Rabelais, a style defined by its robust humor, extravagant use of caricature, bold naturalism, and remedial value.[71] It is likely that Osler deliberately misquoted the Bible (the correct spellings are "Phinehas" and "Eleazar," and the passage is in Numbers [25:7-15], not Exodus) in order to make his protagonist all the more believable as a busy backwoods physician.[72]

From this beginning, Egerton Yorrick Davis cropped up repeatedly in case reports and letters to the editor in medical journals. Osler's students and admirers continued the prank after his death, and indeed "EYD" continues to sneak into the medical literature. When Osler signed his notes EYD his friends knew that he was using the impish or Rabelaisian side of his personality. Thus when the great medical illustrator Max Brödel drew a cartoon of Osler as "The Saint—Johns Hopkins Hospital" in 1896, Osler wrote a caption on a reproduction of the picture: "For this scandalous canonization, & with the consent & approbation of Cardinal Gibbons, Max Brödel is responsible. EYD." [73] Osler often signed hotel registers as "Dr. E. Y. Davis and Mrs. Osler." If a stranger approached and asked whether he was "the famous Dr. Osler," he might say, "No, E. Y. Davis of Caughnawauga, often mistaken for him." [74] Once as Osler was standing on a railway platform in Boston's Back Bay with two other physicians, a man approached him and asked, "Isn't this Dr. Osler?" He replied, "I am Dr. Davis, and these are my friends, Dr. Bigelow and Dr. Ware." Bigelow and Ware were famous Boston physicians from a previous era.[75] These and other escapades may seem inappropriate to us, and perhaps they were. Osler, like most people who are largely free of their inhibitions, had little or no sense of timing and judgment and was sometimes frivolous.[76]

But his practical jokes can be best understood as an attempt to lighten life's burdens—his own and those of others. Perhaps Clifford Allbutt put it best when he noted that "much of his playfulness and whimsical mystification were in the naturalist's phrase, 'a protective colouring' that covered deep sensibilities." [77] When a patient seemed terminally ill or had died and been covered by a shroud, Osler would often walk away whistling. If pressed for a reason, he would say that "I whistle that I may not weep." [78] Conversant as he was with Scripture, he was no doubt familiar with the passage from Proverbs (14:13) that "even in laughter the heart is sorrowful." [79] Osler's "peculiar mixture of foolishness and thoughtfulness" explains, at least in part, why he was so uniformly beloved by his contemporaries and so effective in dealing with patients. His humor kept him from taking himself too seriously. It was an essential part of his capacity to care.

CARE FOR THE RIGHT REASONS

We are left with the issue of the nature and extent of Osler's caring. Let us begin by defining some terms. The vocabulary of caring entails subtle differences between *beneficence, empathy, sympathy,* and *compassion. Beneficence* (from the Latin *beneficentia,* meaning "active kindness") means doing good and is a principle of medical ethics. The physician must respond positively to three questions: What is wrong with the patient? What can I do for the patient? What will be the outcome? *Empathy* (from the Greek *en,* "in," and *pathos,* "feeling") involves understanding the patient's feelings, at least intellectually, in order to be helpful.[80] *Sympathy* (from the Greek *sympatheia,* "like-feeling" or "fellow-feeling") requires that we not only understand but also experience feelings similar to the patient's. *Compassion* (from the Latin *com,* "with," and *passus,* past participle of *pati,* "to suffer") goes one step further: we experience distress to the extent that we actually suffer *with* the patient. Was Osler compassionate in this strict sense of the term? We don't know.[81]

To be sure, many people would rank Osler among the most compassionate of physicians based on actual cases. There were, for example, his relationships with the aging poet Walt Whitman, who suffered from depression, and the great surgeon William S. Halsted, who never completely recovered from addiction to narcotics caused by experiments on himself before the dangers were fully known.[82] In both instances, he cared appropriately, confidently, and confidentially under difficult circumstances. One might also cite Osler's clear statement about empathy to medical students:

> The motto of each of you as you undertake the examination and treatment of a case should be "put yourself in his place." Realize, so far as you can, the mental state of the patient, enter into his feelings. . . . Scan gently his faults. The kindly word, the cheerful greeting, the sympathetic look. . . . [83]

Moreover, his sympathy was evident in his reluctance to give patients a bad prognosis—sometimes to the consternation of the general practitioners who had referred patients to him.[84] As he put it:

> It is a hard matter, and really not often necessary (since Nature usually does it quietly and in good time), to tell a patient that he is past all hope. As Sir Thomas Browne says, "It is the hardest stone you can throw at a man to tell him that he is at the end of his tether"; and yet, put in the right way to an intelligent man it is not always cruel. . . . Our inconsistent attitude is, as a rule, the outcome of the circumstances that of the three factors in practise, heart, head, and pocket, to our credit, be it said, the first named is most potent.[85]

On the other hand, Osler occasionally dismissed patients in ways that strike us today as inappropriate or even condescending. There was, for example, the time a nervous woman, crying in her bed, said, "Oh, Dr. Osler you misjudge me cruelly." Osler, in a serious tone but with a twinkle in his eye, replied: "Madam, I learned early in life never to *judge* any woman and that rule I have strictly kept. Therefore, I cannot have *misjudged* you. Good morning." [86] He seems to have cared the most when his caring was most likely to affect the outcome.

Osler never claimed to be compassionate in the sense of being a "fellow sufferer." Cushing observed, "Almost never did Osler betray his deeper feelings by any show of sentiment. His friends were well aware of this." [87] A student wrote that it "was hard to think of him as a sympathetic human being, able to help us cope with our difficulties and embarrassments in daily life," but that "every one of us has gone to him with our common troubles and he helped us as a man with a warm heart, and for that too, we loved him." [88] Perhaps Osler didn't say much about "compassion" because it is a suspect word, a difficult commodity to verify and impossible to measure. The extent to which Osler was obviously loved by patients, peers, and students illustrates that we are valued less by what we say than by what we do. The physician's first duty is to be competent at what he or she professes to be able to do, and to do it consistently and well. In a sense, acts of benevolent competence *are* compassion, while compassion without competence is fraud. For no amount of "caring" compensates for failure to do what we say we can and will do.

Osler's manner of caring also illustrates that we must care from the context of a healthy personality. If we believe that caring for others will help us feel better about ourselves, we are in store for disappointment, frustration, and even codependency. Aristotle, in *The Nicomachean Ethics*, spoke of the "pleasure of beneficence" and considered it not at all paradoxical that "benefactors . . . love those they have benefited, more than those who have been well treated love those that have treated them well." [89] The explanation lies in basic psychology. When we do good for someone, that person becomes for us the incarnation of our own goodness. We feel better about ourselves and warmly toward our beneficiary. But the beneficiary, whose self-esteem was probably damaged by whatever required our help in the first place, may not reciprocate our warm feelings. The recipient may view our help as nothing special, a mere technical service, and may even sue if things don't turn out well.

To care for the right reasons, we must begin by caring for ourselves and by asking whether the outcome of our caring matters for our own self-esteem. High self-esteem, that emotional sine qua non for happiness, can be recognized both by the presence of such phenomena as sustained success, long-term relationships, frequent affirmation of others, resilience from setbacks, and ability to laugh at oneself and also by the absence of such phenomena as envy, boasting, and criticism of others. William Osler showed these emblems of high self-esteem in abundance. He also knew that lasting self-esteem seldom results from recognition by others. Thus when he was knighted in 1911, he said, "This thing cannot make us any happier, and as we were very contented before, I hope it will not disturb our *Aequanimitas*." [90] When asked whether he preferred "Sir William" or "just plain Dr. Osler," he would usually answer "just plain Dr. Osler." When the question was put to him obnoxiously on one occasion, he immediately quoted from Lewis Carroll's *The Hunting of the Snark*: "I answer to hi or to any loud cry." [91] By keeping his self-esteem at a healthy level and combining it with humility, he was able to help others feel good about themselves, which was an important aspect of his caring.

Although the basis of self-esteem is poorly understood, it is clear that much of it comes from early childhood. Osler was fortunate in at least two ways, the first of which was by accident of birthday. The settlers of Bond Head, Ontario, included a great

	Can control	**Cannot control**
Act	**Mastery**	**Futility**
Don't act	**Surrender**	**Serenity**

Figure 6.1. Effects of acting or not acting, depending on whether or not things are within our control.

many Ulster Scots whose custom it was to celebrate July 12 with an Orange Day parade commemorating the victory of King William III at the Battle of the Boyne. When the merry band reached Parson Osler's house and met the newborn son, they insisted on the name William rather than Walter Farquhar as his parents had planned. The fuss made over "William, the young Prince of Orange" at subsequent parades caused the other children to think that the festivities were a birthday party arranged especially for him![92] Second and more important, he seems to have been the darling of his mother, Ellen Free Pickton Osler, a remarkable woman whose love made him feel (if Freud was correct) invincible.

But if Osler acquired much of his self-esteem in early childhood, he also practiced behaviors now recommended by leading psychologists. Nathaniel Branden, founder of the Branden Institute for Self-Esteem, suggests that we can enhance self-esteem by sticking to our principles, living in day-tight compartments, working toward goals, committing ourselves to lifelong learning, and accepting responsibility for our actions and happiness.[93] Harry Levinson, founder of the Levinson Institute, suggests that we can enhance self-esteem through realistic expectations that minimize the gap between ego ideal (what we would like to be) and self-image (what we think we are).[94] Osler also valued self-awareness, recommending "the advice of Descartes, that everyone should have one examination of himself in his life, a carefully carried out inquisition. . . . Make it searching, make it real, and may it influence your life as much as it did that of the great philosopher." [95] Following such advice today would mean knowing one's psychological makeup and considering counseling to make sure that one is indeed caring for the right reasons and within one's capabilities.[96]

In summary, Osler sought to care in such a way as to be most helpful. He tended to heed the advice of the Stoic philosophers, famously restated by Reinhold Niebuhr in the "Serenity Prayer," that we should act when we can change the outcome but accept things as they are when we cannot (see Figure 6.1).[97] By caring from within the context of a healthy personality and by setting limits, Osler helped others in ways that were specific and straightforward. He did not talk about "compassion" per se, but he was sympathetic, effective at psychotherapy, and usually offered common-sense advice that patients could follow.[98] His style of caring may not be appropriate for everyone but it illustrates the value of finding ways to care that are useful and sensitive yet realistic and within one's capacity. For Osler, the essence of caring was love of craft combined with love of humanity—the Hippocratic ideal for which he stood beyond everything else.

7

COMMUNICATE

Secrets of the Heart

Like most widely influential people, Osler was a great communicator who used language to reach the hearts and minds of others. He is best remembered for his inspirational addresses, but he was also a good classroom teacher, a good committee member, a good host, a good listener, and a good friend. He was not a politician in the strict sense, but he respected the political process and used it when necessary. And he recognized that words can cause unintentional injury and must therefore be chosen carefully.

LEARN TO WRITE

Osler's reputation during his life rested on the quality of his work and the impact of his personality. But as one contemporary predicted, "The memories of the winsome personality of Dr. Osler will pass away, his spoken word is no longer heard, but the written and printed thoughts remain, and upon them will rest the future reputation of Sir William Osler. And fortunate it is that these words are many and of a character worthy of the great man that we knew in the living flesh." [1] His works include numerous editions of his textbook, several monographs, and some 1200 articles in medical journals— a body of literature so vast that it is unlikely that anyone has ever read it all.[2] There was nothing mysterious about how he became an accomplished writer. He had something to say, he studied great writers, he wrote regularly, and he paid meticulous attention to his writing.[3] In short, he worked at it.

Osler's scientific writing was straightforward and concise. Consider the plain but interesting sentence structure of a randomly chosen passage from his textbook of medicine:

> Pain is perhaps the most constant and distinctive feature of [peptic] ulcer. It varies greatly in character; it may be only a gnawing or burning sensation, which is particularly felt when the stomach is empty, and is relieved by taking food, but the more characteristic form comes on in paroxysms of the most intense gastralgia, in which the pain is not only felt in the epigastrium, but radiates to the back and to the sides.[4]

His inspirational essays bring a different kind of pleasure, likened by one critic to "the pleasant movement of a gondola over a Venetian lagoon." [5] His references to history and literature seem almost effortless. And he mastered the use of classical allusions, as illustrated by the opening paragraph of his 1914 address "The War and Typhoid Fever":

> From the days of Homer, Apollo, the far darter, has been a much more formidable foe than his colleague Mars. With the two in conjunction unspeakable woes afflict the sons of men. In his great strait David, you remember, chose three days of pestilence as the equivalent of three months' military disaster. To-day the front of Mars is wrinkled, the world is at war, and the problem for the children of Aesculapius is to keep grandfather Apollo from taking a hand in the fray. In this game another member of the family, Hygeia, holds the trump card and gives victory to the nation that can keep a succession of healthily efficient men in the field. The [British]

Empire is confronted with a great task, in the successful performance of which the medical profession may play a leading part.[6]

Osler's frequent use of classical and literary allusions may strike
today's readers as intellectual overkill. To those who knew him,
however, this style was neither overbearing nor pretentious but
rather flowed naturally from his easy familiarity with his sources.
Despite changing tastes, his essays exude the charm and versatility
of an excellent writer.

Most of Osler's writing was expository, designed to teach rather
than to entertain. He did not seek a literary career outside of
medicine, although he admired those who did, such as Boston's
Oliver Wendell Holmes: "With an entire absence of nonsense, with
rare humour and unfailing kindness, and with that delicacy of
feeling characteristic of a member of the Brahmin class, he has
permanently enriched the literature of the race." [7] Osler seldom
attempted so-called creative writing unless one considers the Egerton Yorrick Davis stories to be of that genre. However, he knew
how to build verbal images and metaphors when the occasion
called for them, as shown by his concluding remarks at an address
he gave in 1911 at the opening of the new Pathological Institute
of the Royal Infirmary in Glasgow:

> The most vivid recollections of my boyhood in Canada cluster about
> the happy spring days when we went off to the bush to make maple
> sugar—the bright sunny days, the delicious cold nights, the camp
> fires, the log cabins, and the fascinating work tapping trees, putting
> in the birch-bark spouts, arranging the troughs, and then going from
> tree to tree collecting in pails the clear, sweet sap. One memory
> stands out above all others, the astonishment that so little sugar was
> left after boiling down so great a cauldron of liquid. And yet the sap
> was so abundant and so sweet. The workers of my generation in the
> bush of science have collected a vaster quantity of sap than ever
> before known; much has already been boiled down, and it is for you
> of the younger generation while completing the job to tap your own
> trees. . . . It is for you in this new infirmary and in this splendid
> institute to see that the quality is maintained.[8]

But for all of his carefully crafted prose, Osler is best remembered for his aphorisms. Many of these pithy encapsulations of
clinical wisdom still reverberate through hospital corridors and

clinics around the world. Generations of medical students and physicians have delighted in such gems as

> Know syphilis in all its manifestations and relations, and all other things clinical will be added unto you.

> Soap and water and common sense are the best disinfectants.

> Man should go out of this world as he came in—chiefly on milk.

> Reasoning from the urine is as brittle as the urinal.

> The normal man walks by faith, the tabetic [a person with syphilis of the spinal cord] by sight.

> Jaundice is a disease that your friends diagnose.

> The chief function of the consultant is to make a rectal examination that you have omitted.[9]

As one contemporary put it:

> Not one of all the thousands who came under his influence but can recall some epigrammatic utterance—some suggestive saying, never to be forgotten but treasured among the priceless memories of cherished associations. In this category belongs his comment on "the advantages of a small amount of albumin in the urine," and his appropriate resurrection of the aphorism for all mouth-breathers, "Shut your mouth and save your life." [10]

Osler's aphorisms convey the image of a master teacher who knew his stuff, liked what he did, and made learning fun.

His writing was not always so memorable. His first medical articles were routine case reports.[11] But he kept on writing and his writing improved, illustrating the truism that "the only way for the average man to learn how to write is to write." [12] As a young faculty member at McGill he volunteered to edit the clinical and pathological reports of the Montreal General Hospital, a job that most people would consider a thankless task. Writing out autopsy reports helped him hone the ability to express himself succinctly. For example:

> William B., æt. 63, a large, powerfully built man, carpenter by trade, was admitted into the Hospital Sept. 18th, complaining of cough and dyspnœa. Has been a healthy man, accustomed all his life to hard work, and until about two years ago had drunk freely. In

October, 1877, caught cold from wearing wet clothes, and was off work for five weeks. In May was laid up with cough, and had, at the same time, swelled feet. Was in Hospital for five weeks. Has worked continuously since that time until the 12th of September, when he had to give up on account of the shortness of breath and swelled feet.[13]

Regular preparation of such straightforward if pedestrian reports also helped him overcome writer's block and submit many articles to medical journals. He urged students to follow his example: "When you have made and recorded the unusual or original observation, or when you have accomplished a piece of research in laboratory or ward, do not be satisfied with a verbal communication at a medical society. Publish it." [14] He was paraphrased as having said, "Avoid carrying unpublished knowledge to the grave." [15] However, he urged quality above quantity: "The young physician should be careful what and how he writes." [16] Moreover, "The difficulty is that the young write too much, the mature write too little. There is too much green fruit sent to market, and the fruit of too many of the fine trees is never plucked at all." [17] Osler had a writer's natural interest in words: "After all, there is no such literature as a Dictionary." [18] He knew that the essence of good writing is revision: "It is often harder to boil down than to write." [19] Scrupulous about his own writing, he became a good editor and proofreader.[20] Finally, he recognized that writing is serious business for the "worth of a book, as of a man, must be judged by results." [21]

Through practice and study, aided by his habit of reading with a notebook and pen at hand, Osler ultimately developed "the charm of style which characterized his later essays." [22] His mature style reflects the influence of many great writers. He was influenced especially by Shakespeare, whom he called "the greatest of the world's creators," and Francis Bacon, "the first of the modern transmuters." [23] Osler's first book purchase, in 1867, was a copy of the Globe Shakespeare, and he quoted Shakespeare not only in his essays but also in his letters. His medical writings contain numerous paraphrasings of Shakespeare. For example, reviewing the issue of when to recommend exploratory surgery, Osler wrote, "But desperate cases require desperate remedies"— similar to Shakespeare's "Diseases desperate grown, / By desperate appliances are relieved / or not at all" (*Hamlet*, act 4, scene 2).[24] Osler wrote that "the Alchemy of Shakespeare made him a great creator. 'Self-school'd, self-scann'd, self-honour'd, self-secure,' in heaven-sent moments he turned the common thoughts of life into gold." [25] He spoke of the need for "a heightened appreciation of the value of Shakespeare in the education of the young." He observed that each generation must discover for itself the timeless truths about humanity that permeate Shakespeare's writings:

> In life's perspective we seniors are apt to resent that the rising generation should work out its own salvation in ways that are not always our ways, and with thoughts that are not always our thoughts. One thing is in our power, to admix in due proportions with their present somewhat rickety bill of fare the more solid nourishment of the English Bible and of Shakespeare.

Francis Bacon was a contemporary of Shakespeare and a writer of such ability that efforts have been made from time to time to assign to him authorship of the plays attributed to Shakespeare. Bacon's moral character and reputation were somewhat mixed. Osler remarked that the "singularly human admixture of greatness and littleness was in his works as well as in his life." Moreover, "Darkly wise and rudely great, Bacon is a difficult being to understand. Except the *Essays*, his books make hard reading." [26] Yet Osler obviously admired Bacon's mastery of the epigram and sometimes even paraphrased him. Thus when he said that "it is easier to buy books than to read them and easier to read them than to absorb them," [27] he echoed Bacon's advice that "some books are to be tasted, others to be swallowed, and some few to be chewed and digested." [28] Osler's mature writing also mirrored his love for Scripture, for the great writers of Greece and Rome, for the other authors on his bedside reading list for medical students, and for good literature in general. But his eventual style was his own.

Osler's writing has attracted many admirers over the years. Edward N. Brush remarked that "a beauty of literary style almost inevitably results" from such "a man who has ideals and honesty of purpose [and] has filled his mind with the productions of the master spirits of the ages." [29] Francis R. Packard wrote:

> Although the writings of Osler abound with quotations from or references to all of those mentioned in his bedside list as well as many other of the classics of literature, yet his literary style is peculiarly his own and his thought untrammelled by bondage to any particular master. It has not the pompous solemnity of the Elizabe-

than prose with which he was so familiar, nor the involved and often obscure phraseology of his beloved Sir Thomas Browne, nor the splendid pomp of Milton's prose which he so often quotes, nor the antithetical accuracy of Addison's. Osler had absorbed all that was best in English literature, both old and new, and as his thoughts were peculiarly his own, the result of his keen observation and logical accuracy, so he expressed them in a clear, lucid and forceful manner, not borrowing his manner of expression from any of the great masters of that art who had preceded him.[30]

Osler would have said that in writing, as in everything else, he succeeded because of method and hard work. He became a versatile and effective writer by combining diligence with a high sense of purpose.

LEARN TO LISTEN

Osler was an effective speaker, but he was probably even more effective as a listener. He taught that listening lies at the core of clinical medicine: "Listen to the patient, he is telling you the diagnosis." [31] A student recalled his parting advice: "Remember silence is golden; don't you do the talking; you do the listening and you'll learn much." [32] Another of his aphorisms reads, "Look wise, say nothing, and grunt. Speech was given to conceal thought." [33] But he grasped that the main purpose of listening is not to conceal one's own thoughts but rather to affirm others by showing interest in them. Osler's enormous popularity among his contemporaries was undoubtedly due in large measure to his ability to listen. Thayer observed that Osler "was a good listener and had an unusual skill in guiding a conversation. If the conversation took a turn of which he disapproved, he could cut it short or change the subject with ease." [34]

But he did not dominate conversations. Edith Reid noted, "He was not a teller of good stories; he rarely told an anecdote; he was not overinterested in hearing one, and never in hearing three or four. His jest was a quick rapier thrust—with the button on—at your frailties, or else an out-and-out practical joke." [35] Photographs of Osler in group settings usually indicate open body language. His eyes are focused on the speaker. His head is often slightly tilted, and his chin likely to rest on his hand. He has good posture, and he seldom folds his arms across his chest or behind his head in such a way as to suggest defensiveness or power. Hiram Woods understood "Osler's motive force: aim to realize the other man's point of view and his needs, and to reach these needs if he could." [36] These observations suggest that he practiced many if not all of the recommendations of today's authorities on listening, who remind us that it is an active process requiring that we absorb, process, and interpret both the verbal and the nonverbal content of what is being said.

Although Osler's ability to listen arose naturally from his interest in other people, it was no doubt reinforced by his perusal of the great minds of the past. What is now called active or attentive listening can be traced to antiquity. Consider, for example, the following selections from Osler's recommended bedside reading list for medical students:

> A wise man will hear, and will increase learning, and a man of understanding shall attain unto wise counsels. (Proverbs 1:5)

> Fix your thought closely on what is being said, and let your mind enter fully into what is being done, and into what is doing it. (Marcus Aurelius, *Meditations*, book 7 [30])

> Be mostly silent; or speak merely what is needful, and in few words. . . . If you are able, then, by your own conversation, bring over that of your company to proper subjects. (Epictetus, *The Enchiridion* [33])

> For my part, answer'd Don *Quixote*, I will hear you attentively. (Cervantes, *Don Quixote*, part 1, book 4, chapter 23.

These remarks reflect the truism that ideas and knowledge seldom enter the mind through an open mouth.

Another author on Osler's reading list, Plutarch, even captured the essence of the active listening process as now understood and taught in a remarkable essay written for the benefit of a teenager named Nicander. Plutarch began by pointing out that "most people go about the matter in the wrong way: they practise speaking before they have got used to listening, and they think that speaking takes study and care, but benefit will accrue from even a careless approach to listening." [37] He went on to describe most if not all of the components of what we now call active listening. Consider, for example, a model known as CARESS—an acronym for concentrating, acknowledging the speaker, researching the speaker's views by asking questions and responding, exercising emotional control, sensing both the verbal and the nonverbal content, and structuring the message in order to make the best use of it.[38] As the following excerpts show, Plutarch covered each of these components:

1. *Concentrate* on the speaker and the substance (not the style) of the message, blocking out distractions including one's own prejudices:

   Anyone who fails to concentrate on the actual topic . . . might as well refuse to drink medicine unless the cup has been made out of Attic clay [a famous pottery clay] . . . such a person . . . is suffering from the diseases which have caused a dearth of intelligence, for the most part, and of good sense, and have filled the schools with pedantry and verbosity.

2. *Acknowledge* the speaker by showing genuine interest:

   Listen to the speaker in a gracious and civilized manner. . . . When the speaker hits the mark, one should acclaim his skill; and one should applaud at least his intention in making public what he knows and in using the arguments he himself has found convincing to try to persuade others.

3. *Research* the speaker's message by asking questions for clarification, and *respond* appropriately and maturely:

   Slant one's questions toward the speaker's expertise or natural ability—those matters in which he excels himself. . . . People who make demands of a speaker which neither nature nor training have equipped him to answer, and who reject and refuse what the speaker has to offer . . . are earning a reputation for bad manners and troublemaking.

4. *Exercise emotional control*, allowing the speaker to finish before interjecting one's own sentiments:

   There are . . . no exceptions to the rule that for a young man silence is undoubtedly an ornament; and never more so than if he listens to someone else without getting worked up and barking out a riposte but—even if the comments are distinctly unwelcome—puts up with them and waits for the speaker to finish and, once the speaker *has* finished, instead of immediately answering back, leaves an interval.

5. *Sense both verbal and nonverbal content* and—when possible—
   show empathy through appropriate body language:

   > Some people think that the speaker has a function, while the
   > listener does nothing. . . . In fact, however, even a guest at a party
   > has a function to perform, if he has good manners; and someone
   > attending a lecture has even more of a function, because he is a
   > shareholder in the speech and a colleague of the speaker. . . .
   > There is a certain harmonious rhythm on both the speaker's and
   > the listener's part, if each of them makes sure that his own conduct
   > is appropriate.

6. *Structure the message,* indexing the key points in such a way as
   to make use of it:

   > When we have left the lecture and are on our own, we can take
   > something which we think the speaker coped with poorly or inade-
   > quately, and make an attempt at the same thing, and put ourselves
   > in the position of trying to remedy, as it were, deficiency x, or to
   > correct fault y, or to express z in a different way. . . . It is not
   > difficult . . . to repudiate a speech once it has been delivered;
   > but it is extremely hard work to raise an improved version instead.

Plutarch concluded that "proper listening is the foundation of
proper living."

It is remarkable and unfortunate that listening seldom receives
such systematic attention in the public schools nearly two millen-
nia since Plutarch wrote "On Listening" for Nicander. Skill at
listening explains in no small way how people such as William
Osler are able to understand, influence, and affirm others. Osler
seemed to be as eager to hear the ideas of his medical students as
he was to tell them his own.[39] He seemed to listen closely to his
patients with extra care when he perceived a special need. There
was, for example, the case of a widow with many poorly explained
symptoms who had been left with seven children and much prop-
erty but little income. He visited her every day while she was in the
hospital and asked questions about the children and the farm to
the extent that "his intensely human interest in her case did more
to build up her morale than buckets of medicine would have."[40]
Osler understood the truism that listening requires effort but
honors the speaker with unspoken respect, concern, and—yes—
love.

LEARN TO SPEAK

It was usually held that Osler's addresses were more impressive in print than in person despite the image, as we read them many decades later, of a polished platform speaker. He was a popular speaker but no orator. One contemporary described him as "wholly simple and devoid of circumstance or of the least attempt at studied eloquence or theatrical effect." [41] As another put it, he "spoke quietly, but very impressively; his language was concise and clearly arranged." [42] And like most people, Osler had to overcome fears of public speaking even to speak at all.

In 1899 he spoke at McGill and recalled his experience 25 years earlier when "this Faculty, with some hardihood, selected a young and untried man to deliver the lectures on the Institutes of Medicine." He confessed that his first efforts, like those of nearly all fledgling speakers, were fraught with anxiety:

> One recollection is not at all shadowy—the contrast in my feelings to-day only serves to sharpen the outlines. My first appearance before the class filled me with a tremulous uneasiness and an overwhelming sense of embarrassment. I had never lectured, and the only paper I had read before a society was with all the possible vaso-motor accompaniment. With a nice consideration my colleagues did not add to my distress by their presence, and once inside the lecture room the friendly greeting of the boys calmed my fluttering heart, and, as so often happens, the ordeal was most severe in anticipation. [43]

Osler won the students over not by brilliance but by obvious careful preparation and delivery stemming from concern that they learn the material. One student recalled, "To any one who merely dropped in for one lecture, Osler's delivery might be described as stumbling, even stuttering, but to us students he was delightfully clear, distinct and convincing." [44] Another student mentioned Osler's "habit of walking up and down the platform. . . . He did not speak volubly, but every word and sentence were well thought out before being said, and so his lectures were very impressive and his teaching deposited deeply and permanently in the recesses of his listeners' brains." [45] A third student seems to have spoken for the entire class:

> Quick and active, yet deliberate in his walk and manner, with a serious and earnest expression, it was evident that he looked upon

his lectures as serious, and at once imparted the same feeling to others. In a very few words he welcomed his class, stated what he hoped to do and what he expected in return, concluding with a gentle warning that he expected attendance and attention from all. We succumbed to that genial and kindly manner which has been so characteristic throughout his life, and I doubt if any professor had more carefully studied lectures, or better attention than was given to him.[46]

The McGill students were understandably dismayed when in 1884 Osler left Montreal for Philadelphia.

Osler never became eloquent in the sense of having "superior oratorical powers." [47] But he was eloquent in two more important ways: conciseness and being *present* for his audiences. As Emerson put it: "It is not powers of speech that we primarily consider under this word *eloquence*, but the power that being present, gives them their perfection, and being absent, leaves them a merely superficial value. Eloquence is the appropriate organ of the highest personal energy." [48] This distinction quickly became apparent to the students at the University of Pennsylvania, who found their new professor from Canada to be, as Cushing put it,

> this swarthy person with drooping moustache and informal ways, who instead of arriving in his carriage, jumped off from a street-car, carrying a small black satchel containing his lunch, and with a bundle of books and papers under his arm; who was apt to pop in by the back door instead of by the main entrance; who wore, it is recalled, a frock-coat, top hat, a flowing red necktie, low shoes, and heavy worsted socks which gave him a foreign look; who, far from having the eloquence of his predecessor, was distinctly halting in speech; who always insisted on having actual examples of the disease to illustrate his weekly discourse on Fridays at eleven, and, as likely as not, sat on the edge of the table swinging his feet and twisting his ear instead of behaving like an orator—this at least was not the professor they had expected.[49]

Some of the more cynical suggested that Osler's halting delivery was an affectation acquired in England. But, as one recalled, "Very soon we forgot all about his manner of speech and realized that he was a man tremendously interested in medicine as a natural science . . . indeed in our opinion he already knew pretty much all that was knowable, and wished most earnestly to make us interested in learning for ourselves." [50] Another remembered: "Little we could afford to lose, for the words that fell from his lips were pearls of wisdom. He was an inspiration, with the faculty of exciting the best in others, and an infinite capacity for taking pains, the true measure of great genius." [51] George Dock, who admired Osler's directness and conversational tone, found it amusing that Osler himself expressed admiration for another professor's "silver tongued" lectures.[52]

The record suggests that Osler steadily honed his ability to reach the hearts and minds of others. In Baltimore the surgeon J. M. T. Finney observed that while Osler was

> exhorting his students, he is at the same time revealing the innermost secrets of his heart. He is telling the secret of his great success, the reason why he was able to accomplish the wonderful work that he did, and how it was that he gained the pinnacle of fame which was his. Yes, Dr. Osler was pre-eminently a teacher. He would have made a wonderful preacher.[53]

Thayer found inspiration in Osler's use of language:

> His talks in the wards were replete with epigrams. The right adjective, often quaint and unusual, was always on the tip of his tongue, and to a rare degree he possessed the power to inspire in the patient confidence, courage, and hope; in the student, enthusiasm.[54]

Another contemporary remembered, "His words were simple, his sentences short, his illustrations apt, and he seemed never at a loss for a reference, a quotation or a happy turn." [55] It is unlikely that any of this happened by accident. Osler was keenly interested in human speech and dialects. Among his unfinished essays was one entitled "The American Voice" and another entitled "The Transatlantic Voice." [56]

He considered speaking a privilege and held that speakers owed it to their audiences to be punctual and concise. He knew that verbosity on a speaker's part trains people not to listen. According to Cushing, "There were two human frailties which perhaps irritated him as much as any others—one of them was unpunctuality, the other was garrulousness; and it was one of his common sayings to students that punctuality and brevity were primary requisitions of a physician and might ensure success even with other qualities lacking." [57] Disliking long-windedness, he once proposed to the Canadian Medical Association that with rare exception papers should be limited to thirty minutes. He said, "It is a miserable mistake . . . to speak for more than half an hour, but to continue for an hour and a quarter is too much for human endurance." [58] He came to realize that audiences nearly always appreciate speakers who have something to say and who say it briefly, however unpolished the delivery might be.

Osler thus succeeded as a speaker because of preparation, practice, enthusiasm for his subject matter, and concern for his audiences. His last major address, "The Old Humanities and the New Science," given in 1919 to the Classical Association of Great Britain, illustrates this point. He revised the lecture many times. He put together two exhibits, one consisting of 20 landmark treatises on medicine and science and the other of early scientific apparatus that he had rounded up in Oxford. The address was "full of learning, of humour, of feeling, of eloquence" and contained "suggestions of real weight with regard to the interconnection of science and the humanities." [59] That Osler would eventually produce such a memorable occasion seems, in retrospect, inevitable. Six years earlier, in 1913, an editorialist had written after one of Osler's addresses:

> One sees now, if he never realized it before, that Dr. Osler would have been great in any field—in the pulpit, in politics, in literature, in journalism, in law—because God gave him a great and exceptional and many-sided mind and a spirit which such minds often lack—the inspiration, the courage and the honesty of the prophet who has walked on the mountain-top and swept the whole world with his eyes, and who can deliver a message that is as unbounded as his vision.[60]

SHARE CONCERNS

Osler multiplied his effectiveness by his ability to relate to the people around him. He may have been stimulated in part by the advice of Sir Thomas Browne that we can learn from everyone:

> For my conversation, it is like the Sun's with all men, and with a friendly aspect to good and bad. I think there is no man bad, and the worst, best; that is, while they are kept within the circle of those qualities wherein they are good: there is no man's mind of such

discordant and jarring a temper, to which a tuneable disposition may not strike a harmony.[61]

Osler's promotion of fellowship, dialogue, and goodwill may have been a natural expression of his personality, but—here again—he succeeded because of planning and priorities. He acknowledged the problem of finding enough time for outside concerns: "In his character as a physician a man has a threefold relation with the public, with the profession and with himself. Not one of us in all, only a few of us in some of these diverse relations, live up to our full capacity." [62] One contemporary noted that "he had a genuine interest in and felt a definite responsibility for the welfare of the community in which he lived." [63]

Osler's ability to relate to people can be broken down into several components. First, he had an uncanny knack for remembering names. Cushing marveled, "It is doubtful if any physician ever had a wider acquaintance among the profession at large, and he had the rare gift of recalling people's names and remembering his associations with them, no matter how brief the previous encounter may have been." [64] He suggested that perhaps Osler's ability with names came from his boyhood at Weston School, where, as head prefect, he was responsible for reciting the school's roll from memory at a moment's notice to determine if any of the pupils were truant. The story of how he greeted Yale students at a tea in 1913 suggests that one of his techniques may have been the use of humorous associations: "He stood at the door to receive them, took each man in turn by the shoulders as he entered and proceeded to give a mock diagnosis of his character." [65] Making funny or colorful mental associations (usually to be kept in private) is now widely recommended as a mnemonic device for remembering names.

Second, he recognized the importance of social functions and made a point of participating (see also Chapter 5). He warned students that lack of social skills could spell professional ruin and said that "I have known instances in which this malady was incurable." [66] Speaking in Philadelphia at the dedication of the Wistar Institute of Anatomy and Biology in 1894, he said of its namesake, Caspar Wistar: "He is its Avicennna, its Mead, its Fothergill, the very embodiment of the physician who, to paraphrase the words of Armstrong, used by Wistar in his Edinburgh Graduation Thesis,

'Sought the cheerful haunts of men, and mingled with the bustling crowd.' " He expanded on this theme:

> Genial and hospitable, he reigned supreme in society by virtue of exceptional qualities of heart and head, and became, in the language of Charles Caldwell, "the *sensorium commune* [common property of those who feel] of a large circle of friends." About no other name in our ranks cluster such memories of good fellowship and good cheer, and it stands to-day in this city a synonym for *esprit* and social intercourse. Year by year his face, printed on the invitations to the "Wistar Parties " . . . perpetuates the message of his life, "Go seek the cheerful haunts of men." [67]

Osler himself sought the "cheerful haunts" and was popular wherever he went.

Third, he was flexible in such a way that he could ignore differences of age, social class, and points of view. A visitor to Oxford observed:

> For Osler was a man to whom differences of years meant little. He had a catholicity of social instinct which enabled him to say the right thing to the youngest freshman and to the oldest Don alike. For the moment, he was always of the same age as the man with whom he spoke—not talking down to one or talking up to another, but instinctively taking the other's point of view and being actually interested in the things that absorbed the other's attention.[68]

Osler may have honed this ability by going out of his way to relate to both children and old people, since in both instances one must concentrate especially hard to see another's point of view. In his address to young military physicians, he implied that our own conceits are likely to pose barriers to openness:

> Enjoying the privilege of wide acquaintance with men of very varied capabilities and training, you can, as spectators of their many crotchets and of their little weaknesses, avoid placing an undue estimate on your own individual powers and position. As Sir Thomas Browne says, it is the "nimbler and conceited heads that never looked a degree beyond their nests that tower and plume themselves on light attainments," but "heads of capacity and such as are not full with a handful or easy measure of knowledge think they know nothing till they know all!" [69]

He knew that we must accept people as we find them.

Finally, he worked to create good social environments, knowing that they seldom happen spontaneously. One physician recalled how Osler's ability to bring people together enlivened what would otherwise have been a lonely lunch hour at the Tenth International Medical Congress in Berlin in 1890:

> Catching me by the arm he at once plunged into a lively series of questions as to what I had been doing at the Congress, whom I had met, and how profitable I had found the meetings. . . . By the time we had reached the restaurant only a short distance away, Osler had joined to our happy trio one by one, five other members, each wandering alone, all congenial friends and delighted to have been admitted to our party and thus rescued from the fate of a lonely meal.[70]

Another physician recalled that Osler's home, even before he married, was a focal point for social gathering:

> The social instinct was always strong in him, and his house was a rendezvous for medical men from far and near. It was an open house at luncheon time, and almost any week one might be certain to meet some well-known figure of the American, and often of the European, medical world at his table or at five o'clock tea. But it was not only the masters of the profession to whom he gave a welcome—his door and his table were open to the humblest practitioner who had need of his advice and care. He was always specially interested in younger men of promise, for whom his personal charm and easy geniality, no less than his professional distinction, had an irresistible attraction.[71]

Osler's ability to create a good social environment received an enormous boost when he married Grace Revere Gross (see Chapter 8). She "made his house almost a delightful Club for his friends and in it an inviolable peace and quiet for himself."[72] In Oxford, the Osler home at 13 Norham Gardens became famous as "The Open Arms," a "Mecca for Americans" and others who happened to be visiting.[73] Osler belonged to so many clubs that he has been criticized more recently as a "club man," but clubs as meaningful forums for discussion mattered more during his era than they do today.[74] And despite his membership in many clubs and the comfort of his home surroundings in his later life, Osler's social ambitions remained essentially egalitarian. He appreciated that the essence of good manners is to include people, not exclude them.

In England he made it a point to get to know all of the area's practitioners, many of whom were isolated and overworked and had little professional stimulation in their lives. An Oxford physician recalled: "The joy and freshness that he brought into some of these men's isolated lives ought to be recorded. They worshiped him. One senior practitioner in a country town near confessed to me that when he heard of his death he sat down and wept." [75] Osler seemed to know that being social is important not to promote ourselves but rather to bring light into the lives of others.

BE POLITICAL

Although Osler has been called a medical politician, he seldom sought or campaigned for office. He twice refused the presidency of the Royal Society of Medicine even after being told that his declination was "an unprecedented snub to the premier medical body of the Kingdom." [76] He refused the presidency of the Medical Society of London and resisted invitations to run for major political office, including a seat in the English Parliament.[77] On December 8, 1905, he made what seems to have been his one and only appearance at a political rally. Having been begged to attend, he managed "successfully and gracefully" to avoid further entanglement with a few well-chosen words. His only open campaign for office was a bid for the Lord Rectorship of Edinburgh University, for which he ran unsuccessfully against two professional politicians after being nominated on short notice. The other losing candidate was Winston Churchill, the future prime minister.[78]

Osler's major contribution to medical politics was to make good politics fashionable. Physicians back then were notorious for petty jealousies. When Osler began his medical studies in Toronto, "envy, hatred, and malice" reigned among the city's doctors, and there was marked tension between the city's two medical schools.[79] He determined that his personal policy would be to promote high standards, to neither make nor hear harsh criticisms, and to promote harmony by working behind the scenes. When he arrived in Baltimore, he again found a bitterly divided medical community. His energy, charm, and devotion to high ideals stilled the hostile camps so well that Baltimore became famous as a center of medical excellence. One physician recalled that his influence came "not in argument or controversy but in the force of example, by the way in which he lived his ideals and induced others to share them with him." [80] When he arrived in England, he quickly became "the real though unobtrusive power in British medicine" and in that capacity "quietly gathered round him some younger men to start the Association of Physicians of Great Britain and Ireland." [81] How did Osler become so influential wherever he went? The answers lie in his personality, promotion of goodwill, and dedication to clear-cut, socially desirable goals. As a McGill student put it, "He had a way of ordering without commanding. His spring of affection was of the same dimensions as his fountain of intellect, and they were both immense." [82]

Osler suggested that physicians, like other citizens, have a duty to take part in the political process. Reflecting on the multifaceted career of the great German pathologist Rudolph Virchow, who served as an alderman on Berlin's city council for 22 years, Osler said, "It will be generally acknowledged that in this country [the United States] doctors are, as a rule, bad citizens, taking little or no interest in civic, state or national politics." [83] However, he taught that major involvement in politics distracts successful physicians from their calling:

> The danger in such a man's life comes with prosperity. He is safe in the hard-working day, when he is climbing the hill, but once success is reached, with it come the temptations to which many succumb. Politics has been the ruin of many country doctors, and often of the very best, of just such a good fellow as he of whom I have been speaking. He is popular; he has a little money; and he, if anybody, can save the seat for the party![84]

In 1918 Osler advised members of the Canadian Army Medical Corps:

> A doctor who comes to me with broken nerves is always asked two questions—(It is unnecessary to ask about drink, as to the practiced eye that diagnosis is easy) about Wall St. and politics. It is astonishing how many doctors have an itch to serve in parliament, but for a majority of them it is a poor business which brings no peace to their souls. . . . You cannot serve two masters, and political doctors are rarely successful in either career. There are exceptions. . . . [but] let the average man who has a family to support and a practice to keep up shun politics as he would drinking and

speculation. As a right-living clear-thinking citizen with all the interests of the community at heart the doctor exercises the best possible sort of political influence.[85]

Osler was no doubt familiar with the strong statement that Oliver Wendell Holmes made to a graduating class of medical students in 1871: "I warn you against all ambitious aspirations outside of your profession. . . . Do not dabble in the muddy sewer of politics, nor linger by the enchanted streams of literature. . . . The great practitioners are generally those who concentrate all their powers on their business." [86]

Osler has been criticized from time to time for his reluctance to enter the fray of political combat. Placing great value on personal relationships, he often held back even when events seemed to warrant strong actions. He tried to avoid confrontation and defuse controversy, especially through humor and persuasion.[87] However, "when the time came—and he was a very wise judge of the proper moment—no one was more fearless or more outspoken than he, as more than one of his colleagues may remember." [88] On one occasion, for example, a man had been proposed for membership in the Association of American Physicians, which was then a small organization consisting mainly of leading internists. Osler arose to protest that the man was only "a second-class general practitioner" who did not deserve the honor.[89] On another occasion, he suggested that the American Medical Association find a new secretary since the aging occupant of that position had become incompetent:

Let the quality of mercy be not strained. I stand here and say plainly and honestly before Dr. Atkinson what I and many other members have said behind his back, that he is not an efficient Secretary of this Association, and that we have not found him so. (Hisses, followed by applause.) You may hiss if you will, but I unhesitatingly say that no more important step in advance will be taken by this Association than when it changes its Secretary.

Mrs. Osler shuddered to hear her husband "maligning old Atkinson the Secretary" even though the remarks were accurate.[90] Atkinson was reelected anyway, and Osler made a point of shaking hands with him afterward.

He did not spare public figures when he thought his cause was just. He once lambasted the mayor of Baltimore for the city's public health problems:

> We are sick to death of mayors and first branches and second branches. In heaven's name, what have they done for us in the past? I can tell you what they have done for us in the thirteen years I have been here. To my positive knowledge they have paved two or three streets east and west, and two or three streets north and south, and, by the Lord Harry! I could not point to a single other thing they have done. . . . Give us a couple or three good men and true who will run the city as a business corporation. It would not take us a year, then, Mr. Mayor, not a year, to get a start on a sewerage system and an infectious disease hospital, and everything else that the public welfare demands.

This attack probably helped the cause of public sanitation, and indeed shortly afterward the mayor was seen "with his arm on Osler's shoulder, talking to him in a way that was earnest but also friendly." [91] On another occasion—known in the colorful history of Baltimore politics as the "Marsh Market" affair of 1895, in which poll watchers including Johns Hopkins faculty members were injured while trying to curb "repeater" voting—Osler responded by writing a humorous poem patterned after Keats.[92] His tact was also tried in 1900 at a United States Senate committee hearing on vivisection:

> The blood just surged in my veins, Sir, when I heard two men address you to-day, say things which they should have been ashamed to say of the medical profession, of men who daily give their lives for their fellows. . . . With reference to men who train with these enemies of the profession, I say this, that I scorn them from my heart.[93]

But Osler usually succeeded at separating the people from the issues. William H. Welch observed after Osler's death how effective he had been at addressing political issues:

> Osler was keenly alive to the implications and applications of modern medicine to the problems of society. Speaking with the authority and influence of a commanding reputation, with full knowledge and with rare gifts of vivid expression, he was a great force in arousing professional and public interest in such modern movements as the better care and control of tuberculosis, of typhoid fever, of malaria, of venereal diseases, and in general of improved public health administration. His name is identified especially with the launching of the anti-tuberculosis campaign as a national movement in Amer-

ica, and he continued his activity in this field in Great Britain. He occupied an advanced progressive position and was active in his later years especially in the attack upon some of the most important problems of preventive medicine.[94]

Similarly, the surgeon J. M. T. Finney remarked that although Osler "was never heard to speak ill of any one" he could nevertheless "enter a vigorous protest against some wrong or wrongdoer . . . and at times in truly picturesque fashion." [95] Controlled anger can be especially powerful when it emanates from someone widely known for praise and tolerance, as Osler was. Osler's effectiveness was also enhanced by his ability to measure people, to see through their mannerisms and superfluity. On one occasion, for example, a patient called out to him, "Good morning, Doc." When the man was out of hearing range, Osler turned to his colleague and said, "Beware of the men that call you Doc. They rarely pay their bills." [96]

BE CAREFUL WHAT YOU SAY

As Osler's reputation grew during his Montreal period, other physicians began to consult him on difficult cases. The format for medical consultations was quite different from what we know today. The consulting physician usually examined the patient in the presence of the referring physician. The two doctors then discussed the case first between themselves and then with the patient or the patient's family. On one occasion, Osler saw a patient in consultation for a taciturn older physician and made a correct diagnosis of typhoid fever. When the consultation was over, the older man said to Osler, "Young man, you talk too much. You have told these people more in fifteen minutes than I have in fifteen years." Osler was fond of telling this story on himself and never forgot the lesson.[97]

Whether from that experience or from others, he took pains to measure his speech. As one colleague put it, "He was always slow to give his opinion until he was sure, and then he gave it in a few words." [98] Harvey Cushing put it more strongly: "Osler was a man of action rather than words." [99] Speaking to nurses, Osler made clear the virtue of taciturnity:

Printed in your remembrance, written as headlines on the tablets of your chatelaines, I would have two maxims: "I will keep my mouth shut as it were with a bridle," and "If thou hast heard a word let it die with thee." Taciturnity, a discreet silence, is a virtue little cultivated in these garrulous days when . . . speech has taken the place of thought. As an inherited trait it is perhaps an infirmity, but the kind to which I refer is an acquired faculty of infinite value. Sir Thomas Browne drew the distinction nicely when he said, "Think not silence the wisdom of fools, but, if rightly timed, the honour of wise men, who had not the infirmity but the virtue of taciturnity," the talent for silence Carlyle calls it.[100]

He was aware that words can be hurtful. Thayer thus paraphrased his advice:

Mix with your colleagues; learn to know them. But in your relations with the profession and with the public, in everything that pertains to medicine, consider the virtues of taciturnity. Look out. Speak only when you have something to say. Commit yourself only when you can and must. And when you speak, assert only that of which you know. Beware of words—they are dangerous things. They change color like the chameleon, and they return like a boomerang.[101]

Osler was wary of the news media. He advised physicians to beware what he called the "Delilah of the press":

In the life of every successful physician there comes the temptation to toy with the Delilah of the press—daily and otherwise. There are times when she may be courted with satisfaction, but beware! Sooner or later she is sure to play the harlot, and has left many a man shorn of his strength, viz., the confidence of his professional brethren.[102]

In this vein, he tried to avoid newspaper reporters as best he could. When they came to his house, he would ask his butler, Morris, to tell them, "No, sir, Dr. Osler left for Timbuctoo this afternoon and won't be home till day after tomorrow." When a reporter caught him on his doorstep on one occasion, he replied to the initial question, "Oh, no, I'm not the famous Dr. Osler; that's my father. You must often have seen the old man walking on Charles St. with the Cardinal about five every afternoon." [103] But the reporters eventually got even with him through the notorious "Fixed Period" controversy.

The year was 1905, and the occasion was Osler's farewell address to the faculty of The Johns Hopkins University. Osler was trying to console an audience that did not want to see him go:

> There are several problems in university life suggested by my depar-
> ture. . . . A man may have built up a department and have gained
> a certain following, local or general; nay, more, he may have had a
> special value for his mental and moral qualities, and his fission may
> leave a scar, even an aching scar, but it is not for long. . . . A man
> comes into one's life for a few years, and you become attached to
> him, interested in his work and in his welfare, and perhaps you grow
> to love him, as a son, and then off he goes!—leaving you with a
> bruised heart.[104]

Osler offered two philosophic perspectives on his departure. First, relocations are both normal and healthy for academic persons. Second—and here came the difficulty—he had little more to contribute anyway since at 55 he was well past his prime.

Osler put forth "two fixed ideas well known to my friends, harmless obsessions with which I sometimes bore them, but which have a direct bearing on this important problem." He continued:

> The first is the comparative uselessness of men above forty years of
> age. This may seem shocking, and yet read aright the world's history
> bears out the statement. Take the sum of human achievement in
> action, in science, in art, in literature—subtract the work of the
> men above forty, and while we should miss great treasures, even
> priceless treasures, we would practically be where we are to-day.

The second "fixed idea," the one that got him into trouble, was that men should retire at age 60. Osler's mistake was to allude to one of Anthony Trollope's lesser-known novels, *The Fixed Period*. The plot is set on an imaginary island in the Pacific named Britannula, whose colonists become convinced that most of the world's problems are caused by the elderly. They propose a college called Necropolis where men are retired at the age of 67 for a year of contemplation before committing suicide by the traditional Roman method of exsanguination in a warm bath. Osler's reference to Trollope was brief and, on the key subjects of age and method, inaccurate:

> My second fixed idea is the uselessness of men above sixty years of
> age, and the incalculable benefit it would be in commercial, politi-

cal and in professional life if, as a matter of course, men stopped work at this age. In his *Biathanatos* Donne tells us that by the laws of certain wise states sexagenarii were precipitated from a bridge, and in Rome men of that age were not admitted to the suffrage and they were called *Depontani* because the way to the senate was *per pontem* [through the bridge], and they from age were not permitted to come thither. In that charming novel, *The Fixed Period*, Anthony Trollope discusses the practical advantages in modern life of a return to this ancient usage, and the plot hinges upon the admirable scheme of a college into which at sixty men retired for a year of contemplation before a peaceful departure by chloroform. That incalculable benefits might follow such a scheme is apparent to any one who, like myself, is nearing the limit, and who has made a careful study of the calamities which may befall men during the seventh and eighth decades. . . . The teacher's life should have three periods, study until twenty-five, investigation until forty, profession until sixty, at which age I would have him retired on a double allowance. Whether Anthony Trollope's suggestion of a college and chloroform should be carried out or not I have become a little dubious, as my own time is getting so short.[105]

On this occasion, Osler's penchant for humor and literary allusion proved most unfortunate. Newspapers throughout the United States blared, "OSLER RECOMMENDS CHLOROFORM AT SIXTY." Scores of cartoons, editorials, and letters to editors fueled the flames of ridicule, anger, and resentment. "To Oslerize" became a synonym for committing euthanasia. Holding firm to the idea that most creative work is done before age 60, Osler resisted the pleadings of his friends that he make a public apology. But he hurt inside. His wife called him "the shattered idol." He wrote privately, "I do not believe any one took the trouble to give exactly what I said. . . . The hubbub did a good deal of harm, and I was heartily sorry for the many old people who were hurt by the outcry." [106] Although some of his finest farewell addresses were still to come, his departure from North America had been tainted by unwanted controversy brought about entirely by a sensationalizing press.[107] It was only after he was safely in Oxford that he wrote the next year, when he added the controversial address to the second edition of *Aequanimitas*,

I jokingly suggested for the relief of a senile professoriate an extension of Anthony Trollope's plan mentioned in his novel, *The Fixed*

Period. To one who had all his life been devoted to old men, it was not a little distressing to be placarded in a world-wide way as their sworn enemy, and to every man over sixty whose spirit I may have thus unwittingly bruised, I tender my heartfelt regrets. Let me add, however, that the discussion which followed my remarks has not changed, but has rather strengthened my belief that the real work of life is done before the fortieth year and that after the sixtieth year it would be best for the world and best for themselves if men rested from their labours.[108]

There are several footnotes to this sorry incident. First, Trollope never mentioned chloroform. Second, Osler's remarks may well have been rooted in deep philosophical and religious conviction that stemmed from his close reading of Sir Thomas Browne's *Religio Medici*.[109] Finally, Osler assumed full responsibility for the incident and dealt with the stress in part with his famous sense of humor. He confided to a friend, "The way of a joker is hard. I deserve to have been caught years ago." [110] And reflecting back on his life in 1916, he told young men at Oxford, "Boys, do not read Trollope. He is dangerous." [111]

8

SEEK

BALANCE

A Simple and Temperate Life

In "The Choice," William Butler Yeats wrote, "The intellect of man is forced to choose / Perfection of the life or of the work." As a young man William Osler chose perfection of the work when he set out to rank among the best in his field. Aiming to be the best at anything makes the balanced life a difficult proposition (Figure 8.1). Osler can be faulted for falling short. To concentrate on medicine, he postponed marriage until his early forties with the result that he and his wife felt fortunate to have even one surviving child. His son's death in World War I broke his heart and, many contemporaries believed, contributed to his own death from pneumonia two years later. But in failing to bring perfect balance to his life, William Osler was hardly

187

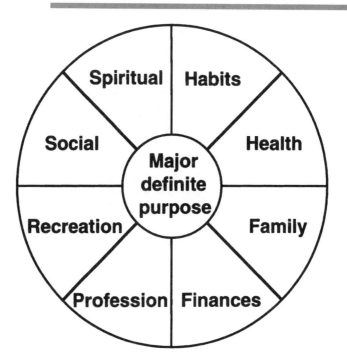

Figure 8.1. The ideal of a balanced life centered on a major definite purpose.

unique. Most of us consider our priorities to be first health, then family, and last job, yet we mete out our waking hours in exactly the reverse order. Still, Osler had much to say about balancing health, marriage and the family, friendships, hobbies, and our common spiritual dilemma. And he died according to his own stated principle, "ready when the day of sorrow and grief came to meet it with the courage befitting a man." [1]

BE A GOOD ANIMAL

Osler urged a simple lifestyle built around mental calmness, sensible habits, and physical activity. He said, "Patients should have rest, food, fresh air, and exercise—the quadrangle of health." [2] He exhorted young physicians, "Live a simple and a temperate life, that you may give all your powers to your profession. Medicine is a jealous mistress; she will be satisfied with no less." [3] He stressed the principles of prevention:

> To each one of us life is an experiment in Nature's laboratory, and she tests and tries us in a thousand ways, using and improving us if we serve her turn, ruthlessly dispensing with us if we do not. Disease is an experiment, and the earthly machine is a culture medium, a test tube, and a retort—the external agents, the medium and the reaction constituting the factors. We constantly experiment with ourselves in food and drink, and the expression so often on our lips, "Does it agree with you?" signifies how tentative are many of our daily actions. [4]

In a lecture titled "The Reserves of Life," he told students,

> Learn early to take the best possible care of the machine, never over-driving it, nor letting rust or dust collect in the bearings, and providing it with enough fuel to keep it going at a fair pace. Unlike any ordinary mechanism, the more you use it, the more, within limits, you can get out of it. Healthy action in a body out of which you can get plenty of work is the first great asset in the race, the most important part, perhaps, of life's reserves. [5]

Osler emphasized the need for a high energy level: "With a fresh, sweet body you can start aright without those feelings of inertia that so often . . . make the morning's lazy leisure usher in a useless day." [6] He was at his most colorful as a temperance advocate, saying, "Who serve the gods die young—Venus, Bacchus, and Vulcan send in no bills in the seventh decade." [7] Venus (goddess of love, hence of sexually transmitted diseases), Vulcan (god of fire and metalworking, hence of heavy labor or possibly of smoking), and Bacchus (god of wine) took their tolls in different ways:

> Vulcan plays with respectability, he allows a wide margin—unless one is a college man—he sends in his bills late in life. Venus is heartless—she sends in her bills throughout all decades. Bacchus is a respecter of persons. North of the Tweed [that is, in Scotland] he may be disregarded—he sends no bills there. [8]

Although Bacchus might respect Scots (for whatever reason), he was still to be feared:

It only too frequently happens that early in the fifth decade, just as business or political success is assured, Bacchus hands in heavy bills for payment, in the form of serious disease of the arteries or of the liver, or there is a general breakdown.[9]

More forcefully:

Throw all the beer and spirits into the Irish Channel, the English Channel, and the North Sea for a year, and people in England would be infinitely better. It would certainly solve all the problems with which the philanthropists, the physicians, and the politicians have to deal.[10]

Abstinence might be the best policy for everyone if only because we cannot predict who is predisposed to alcoholism:

To drink, nowadays, but few students become addicted, but in every large body of men a few are to be found whose incapacity for the day results from the morning clogging of nocturnally-flushed tissues. As moderation is very hard to reach, and as it has been abundantly shown that the best of mental and physical work may be done without alcohol in any form, the safest rule for the young man is that which I am sure most of you follow—abstinence.[11]

Tobacco should also be avoided, at least in excess:

A bitter enemy to the bright eye and the clear brain of the early morning is tobacco when smoked to excess, as it is now by a large majority of students. Watch it, test it, and if need be, control it. That befogged, woolly sensation reaching from the forehead to the occiput, that haziness of memory, that cold fish-like eye, that furred tongue, and last week's taste in the mouth—too many of you know—I know them—they often come from too much tobacco.[12]

Osler promoted sensible diets with such aphorisms as "One pancake for lunch and half a boiled egg for dinner makes a man at sixty able to do anything a college athlete can do" and "We are all dietetic sinners; only a small percent of what we eat nourishes us, the balance goes to waste and loss of energy." [13] He advocated good oral hygiene, "the gospel of cleanliness—cleanliness of the mouth, of the teeth, of the throat." [14] And beyond these specifics, he preached temperance as a general attitude:

Against our third great foe—vice in all its forms—we have to wage an incessant warfare, which is not less vigorous because of the quiet, silent kind. Better than any one else the physician can say the word in season to the immoral, to the intemperate, to the uncharitable in word and deed.[15]

Physicians should therefore teach and model temperance, charity, and morality.

Osler "leaned toward asceticism" in his personal habits. He used alcohol sparingly and was fastidious about what he ate. A Baltimore colleague recalled "how impressed I was with his moderation in the gratification of the physical appetites, and with the regularity of his habits of work and of sleep, indeed with the general *orderliness* of his life." But Osler was no prude. Moderation did not diminish his capacity for fun. He once entered a room where a group of colleagues were enjoying a "night cap" and "insisting that he always took his whiskey 'neat' . . . swallowed—a half a thimble-full!"[16] On another occasion he found himself with a group enjoying oysters and "chose the largest oysters ever seen and then showed great disgust with us that we did not know how to swallow them at a single gulp, so with a readiness which bespoke capacity and capability, as well as delight, he demonstrated how the thing should be done."[17] At a time when the dangers were not fully known, he even smoked.

Osler took an active interest in his own health and made notes on his illnesses.[18] Infectious diseases were the major cause of morbidity and mortality, and he was no stranger to them. He had severe croup as a boy, osteomyelitis of the tibia as a teenager (from playing rugby), smallpox in his twenties (despite having been vaccinated), and recurrent respiratory infections as an older adult. However, he was perhaps ahead of his time in recognizing the extreme importance of atherosclerosis in determining how long we live. He said, "Longevity is a vascular question."[19] Especially after his brother B. B. died of coronary disease at age 61, Osler experienced anxiety about his heart. By age 53, he began to have symptoms that he thought might represent angina pectoris, a disease on which he was an authority. He wrote in his "Autobiographical Notes," which were sealed until 1976, that he had experienced "several days of sub-sternal tension, a warning of too high pressure."[20] In 1917 he dreamed that he was present at his own autopsy:

My own Post-Mortem. Extraordinary dream. . . . Gibson [a pathologist] came up and said to me quietly "You had better not wait

as it may embarrass Allbutt [a clinician and old friend of Osler's]."
I replied "Not a bit. I do not mind. I must see of what he died. Had
he had many attacks?" "No," Gibson said, "only one or two and he
died suddenly last night in a severe angina attack." . . . Gibson
proceeded with the post-mortem, and Allbutt discussed with me
several points about my own case and I told him that years ago I
often had substernal distress which I regarded as the initial step in
the disease. . . . I saw Allbutt and Gibson talking quietly together,
and the former came up and said "You do not mind, Osler, if I report
the case—it can do you no harm as you are really dead. This
appearance of yours is very unusual and quite difficult to explain."
. . . I woke up just as we were going into the histological room to
see the sections of the aorta.[21]

Osler's autopsy two years later showed moderately advanced
atherosclerosis of the coronary arteries, especially of the left ante-
rior descending artery—the branch popularly known among doctors as "the widow-maker." [22]

Osler's basic prescription for health resembled Francis Bacon's:

To be free-minded and cheerfully disposed of meat and of sleep and
of exercise, is one of the best precepts of long lasting. As for the
passions and studies of the mind; avoid envy; anxious fears; anger
fretting inwards; subtle and knotty inquisitions; joys and exhilara-
tions in excess; sadness not communicated. Entertain hopes; mirth
rather than joy; variety of delights, rather than surfeit of them;
wonder and admiration, and therefore novelties; studies that fill the
mind with splendid and illustrious objects, as histories, fables, and
contemplation of nature. . . . I commend rather some diet for
certain seasons, than frequent use of physic, except it be grown into
a custom. . . . In sickness, respect health principally; and in
health, action.[23]

Physical fitness for older adults was not a popular subject during
Osler's lifetime. There is no evidence that he adhered to a routine
of aerobic exercise. Although Osler had been athletic as a young
man—winning flat and hurdle races and holding an unofficial
school record for throwing the cricket ball—he seldom practiced
or preached aerobic exercise for adults. It was mainly through
dietary discretion that he survived numerous banquets and dinner
parties without gaining a great deal of weight. Still, he valued
exercise and thus praised Oxford University for "the way they have

settled the athletic problem. All the men are at exercise in some form, every day, rain or shine, as part of their regular routine." [24] From a lecture he gave to a lay audience on "The Care of the Body" it was gleaned that he had "pleaded for the simple life, with plenty of fresh air and lots of good, hard work as the only means of attaining comfort and peace." [25] And he also said, "A physician who treats himself has a fool for a patient." [26]

HAVE FAMILY

Although Osler came from a large, close-knit family and cherished family ties, he postponed marriage until he was 42. He is often quoted as having said that "medicine is a jealous mistress" and "he travels fastest who travels alone," but it is unlikely that he originated either adage.[27] He did make a strong case to young physicians that they put their passions into "cold storage," as he had done:

> The mistress of your studies should be the heavenly Aphrodite, the motherless daughter of Uranus. Give her your whole heart, and she will be your protectress and friend. A jealous creature, brooking no second, if she finds you trifling and coquetting with her rival, the younger, earthly Aphrodite, daughter of Zeus and Dione, she will whistle you off and let you down the wind to be a prey, perhaps to the examiners, certainly to the worm regret. In plainer language, put your affections in cold storage for a few years, and you will take them out ripened, perhaps a bit mellow, but certainly less subject to those frequent changes which perplex so many young men.[28]

His advice that young nurses should marry, while young physicians should not, seems out of date and suggests a double standard: "Marriage is the natural end of the trained nurse. So truly as a young man marred is a young man married, is a woman unmarried, in a certain sense, a woman undone." [29] His main theme was that youthful passions distract us from our work and tempt us to marry the wrong person.

Osler's recommendation that young physicians should be full-time students was reinforced by the musings of Sir Thomas Browne concerning the dangers of passion:

> I could be content that we might procreate like trees, without conjunction, or that there were any way to perpetuate the world

without this trivial and vulgar way of coition; It is the most foolish act a wise man commits in all his life, nor is there anything that will more deject his cold imagination, when he shall consider what an odd and unworthy piece of folly he has committed; I speak not in prejudice, nor am averse from that sweet sex, but naturally amorous of all that is beautiful.[30]

Osler echoed Browne's conviction that passion makes it hard to concentrate on schoolwork of any kind, warning students of

the heavy burden of the flesh which Nature puts on all of us to ensure a continuation of the species. To drive Plato's team taxes the energies of the best of us. One of the horses is a raging, untamed devil, who can only be brought into subjection by hard fighting and severe training. This much you all know as men: once the bit is between his teeth the black steed Passion will take the white horse Reason with you and the chariot rattling over the rocks to perdition.[31]

Another author on Osler's bedside reading list, Cervantes, made it clear in *Don Quixote* that sexual desire alone seldom assures lasting love:

But as what we call Love in young Men, is too often only an irregular Passion, and boiling Desire, that has no other Object than sensual Pleasure, and vanishes with Enjoyment, while real Love, fixing it self on the Perfections of the Mind, is still improving and permanent.[32]

Osler's favorite literary illustration of the perils of youthful ardor was Tertius Lydgate, the idealistic young surgeon in George Eliot's *Middlemarch* who impetuously marries the beautiful but shallow, materialistic, and strong-minded Rosamond Vincy. Rosamond doesn't care about Lydgate's earnest desire to advance the science and practice of medicine. She wants only the comforts and position of a society doctor's wife, and she gets her wish to Lydgate's misfortune. We may not admire Rosamond, but the fault is Lydgate's for allowing passion to prevail over reason. Osler said, "This well-drawn character in George Eliot's *Middlemarch* may be studied with advantage by the physician; one of the most important lessons to be gathered from it is—marry the right woman!" [33] And he was no doubt reflecting on Rosamond and her ilk when he advised young physicians to "choose a freckle-faced girl for a wife; they are invariably more amiable." [34]

Although Osler did not marry until his fifth decade, he enjoyed a series of close relationships through surrogate families.[35] As a medical student in Montreal he was especially close to two cousins, Marian and Jennette Osler. The former married G. G. Francis, whom Osler knew as "Beelzebub," and named her first son (William W. Francis) after Osler. The boy adored Osler, who was named his godfather. He received a medical degree but retired from active practice after developing tuberculosis and finished out his life as a librarian devoted to William Osler's memory.[36] In addition to such surrogate families, Osler developed a habit of treating many people as family. He often dropped in unexpectedly, bringing a book or flowers for the adults and toys for the children. Cushing referred to these surprise visits as a "pleasant habit," but they were pleasant largely because Osler planned them, fit in with young and old alike, and did not outstay his welcome.[37]

Osler met his future wife in Philadelphia. She had been born Grace Linzee Revere, the great-granddaughter of the American Revolutionary patriot Paul Revere, and her patrician background included refined manners, a keen sense of humor, and a solid social conscience. During a visit to Philadelphia she caught the eye of a surgeon 17 years her senior, Samuel W. Gross, while attending a party. He determined on the spot to marry her. She married him in 1876 despite her family's reservations about the age difference. Earlier that same year Gross had gone to a medical meeting in England and had been so impressed by a young Canadian named William Osler that he suggested to his father, the famous surgeon Samuel D. Gross, that perhaps they could entice him to Philadelphia someday. Eight years later the younger Gross was indeed among those who prevailed on Osler to leave his native Canada. Osler became a close friend of Grace and Samuel Gross, often stopping by their house for dinner or tea. Then in April 1889, Gross developed pneumonia. Before he died, he asked his three physicians to take care of his wife. One of them was Osler, who had already accepted the appointment in Baltimore.

The details of the courtship are largely unknown. It is surmised that Osler proposed on at least one occasion. But he was writing his textbook, and she told him to "stick to his last." Tradition holds that in February 1892 he threw his first copy of the book in her

lap, saying, "There, take the darn thing; now what are you going
to do with the man?" [38] The several people who were told of the
engagement were sworn to secrecy. On the morning of May 7,
1892, Osler took a train from Baltimore to Philadelphia. He and
Grace were sitting in her garden when Dr. James C. Wilson
dropped by and stayed for lunch. Osler nonchalantly reminisced
with Wilson about Canada. Grace, becoming nervous, suggested
that she had to leave as a carriage was waiting for her. Only then
did the friend excuse himself. They were married that afternoon in
St. James Church, Philadelphia, in a service that was apparently
attended by no members of either family. Osler gleefully telegraphed Wilson, "It was awfully kind of you to come to the wedding breakfast." [39]

Mrs. Osler, or "Lady Gross" as he sometimes called her, enhanced his life in numerous ways. Her warm personality and her
previous experience running the Gross household enabled her to
create a gracious yet unpretentious environment where Osler
could entertain as he liked. Their home at One West Franklin
Street in Baltimore became a haven for family, friends, relatives,
colleagues, and medical students. J. M. T. Finney reminisced,
"Many a homesick student will recall with pleasure her gracious
kindness to him, a perfect stranger, and her spontaneous and
genuine cordiality which made him forget himself and feel at once
at home." [40] She encouraged Osler's private consulting practice,
which was necessary since by 1904 she employed a staff of five
servants to help her run the household. At Oxford she helped him
win over a large portion of the university community by sharing his
"real love and interest in everyone." [41] She remained devoted to
Osler after his death, assisting in the cataloguing of his books and
helping in a number of projects to perpetuate his name in what
has been called "the Osler mystique." She did not forget her first
husband, either, and provided in her will that a professorship in
surgery be established at his school, the Jefferson Medical College
of Philadelphia.[42]

If Grace was a superb wife, what kind of husband was William
Osler? A story of Grace's visit to Paris in 1908 suggests that he kept
up a sense of playfulness in the marriage. He had gone ahead of
her and stayed in a mediocre hotel where he was "nearly devoured"
by mosquitoes. Before she came, he found a luxurious apartment
in a better part of town. When Mrs. Osler arrived, he took her to

the unimpressive hotel and apologized that he could not find anything better. He then surrendered the keys, drove off, and swept her into the new quarters, complete with servants, "before she knew that she had been fooled." [43] On the other hand, we can imagine that his gregariousness did not always sit well. She never knew how many people he would bring home for lunch. Indeed, she bought so many groceries that at least one person at Oxford "thought she must be ordering for a hotel." [44] On April 6, 1919, Lady Osler wrote, "What do you think has happened this eve? Sir William and I are having supper alone!!!" [45] And it was she who, after her husband had conveniently left Baltimore just before they were to move to Oxford, was stuck with the details of packing and shipping their household effects across the Atlantic. She was heard to mutter, "Willie's motto may well be Aequanimitas because he always flies when things like this are going on." [46]

Grace Revere Gross was nearly 38 when she married Osler and the likelihood of children therefore uncertain. A first child, Paul Revere Osler, died seven days after his birth. A second pregnancy was complicated by peritonitis during the first trimester. But on December 28, 1895, Grace delivered a seven-pound, blue-eyed boy whom they named Edward Revere Osler. The ecstatic but nervous father waited five days before he kissed him.

Revere, as they called him, was unlike his father in many ways. He was shy and not especially inclined toward either sports or schoolwork. At nine he developed a passion for fishing, and his father nicknamed him Isaac, or Ike, after the great angler Izaac Walton. Subsequent family vacations centered around Revere's fishing expeditions. Revere also took up cabinetmaking and drawing. William Osler tried to interest him in science even to the point of taking a field trip to obtain specimens for examining with the microscope—as Father Johnson had done for him—but it didn't take. Revere eventually showed a love for books and was accepted into Oxford on his second try. Then World War I intervened. Premonitions haunted William and Grace Osler as their son answered the call of duty. On August 29, 1917, as Second Lieutenant E. R. Osler helped move Battery A of the 59th Brigade closer to the front lines with 19 other men, a 4.2–inch German shell exploded in their midst. He died the next morning of chest and abdominal wounds and was buried in Belgium near Poperinghe.[47]

Osler was sitting at his library desk working on a new edition of his textbook when he received the first telegram: "Revere dangerously wounded, comfortable and conscious, condition not hopeless." He wrote in his diary: "I knew this was the end. We had expected it. The Fates do not allow the good fortune that has followed me to go with me to the grave—call no man happy till he dies." [48] He kept up a brave front but never recovered from his grief, confirming that for most of us little if anything ultimately transcends family.

HAVE FRIENDS

If anything soothed Osler during his last years, it was his wife and his many supportive friends. He made friends easily, and it was said of him that he never lost a friend despite changing locations and interests. He kept up with his boarding school chums Ned Milburn and Charlie Locke long after the trio's reputation as "Barrie's bad boys" had been forgotten. Locke became a physician but died young, whereupon Osler assumed responsibility for educating his three children, including putting one of them through medical school.[49] The preserved correspondence between Osler and Milburn, who spent his career as a schoolteacher in Belleville, Ontario, offers a textbook example of how to keep up with old friends.[50] Cushing recalled that memories of their escapades brought Osler some of his greatest pleasures toward the end of his life:

> He would always laugh till the tears came into his eyes at the thought of how "that old pig looked as he rolled over on his back with his four legs stiff in the air," and of how the farmer came out and took him by the scruff of his neck straight home; and his father had to pay eight dollars for the pig. . . . During those last sad years I never saw him laugh so heartily or look so happy as when he forgot the present and lived again his old pranks.[51]

Osler's impish sense of humor always seemed to dwell just below the surface of his demeanor and no doubt helped him win new friends at each stage of life.

Like most lasting friendships, Osler's began with common interests and included a willingness to share old friends with new ones. A student who worked with Osler at McGill Medical School recalled:

> From those who were willing and ready to work with him his demands were unlimited, but for this he more than repaid in the opportunities and good-fellowship that he returned. I thus had every opportunity for the most intimate knowledge of all his mental and physical activities. Soon I found that through his whole-heartedness his friends had become my friends, but not, of course, through any virtue of mine: his pleasures and joys he shared with all those about him, talking freely of all that he had on hand, for in his ebullient enthusiasm he was still a schoolboy.[52]

Another characteristic of Osler's friendships was his generosity. Lewellys F. Barker recalled how Osler's friendships flowed from his love of literature and books:

> How many of us there are who owe to him our introduction to one or another of the great authors of the past—to Plato, to Plutarch, to Burton, to Sir Thomas Browne, or to one or more of his favourite philosophers or poets! And in our own little libraries, what books are more cherished than those that came as gifts from him? I prize my folio Shakespeare the more because of the way it came to me.[53]

His friendships were further facilitated by his cheerfulness, informality, and eagerness to meet people. As one colleague put it:

> Whenever he came into a house an atmosphere of cheerfulness was diffused from him, and people enjoyed being in his company, it was impossible not to feel at your ease with him. He thoroughly loved meeting people and hence was most faithful in his attendance at gatherings of doctors, the more informal they were the better he liked them, the more red tape and ceremony the less happy was he. His perpetual youth endeared him to his friends and acquaintances, he was always cheerful, quick to see humour, tolerant of others however foolish.[54]

Finally, his friendships were marked by persistence as shown by his keeping up with "his old boyhood companions, his teachers, his colleagues, his children, his pupils, and . . . the children of all of them" even from across the sea.[55] His friends mattered.

Osler made clear the priority of friendships when he reminisced about leaving Canada for Philadelphia at age 35:

> After ten years of hard work I left this city a rich man, not in this world's goods, for such I have the misfortune—or the good fortune—lightly to esteem; but rich in the goods which neither rust nor moth have been able to corrupt,— in treasures of friendship and good-fellowship, and in those treasures of widened experience and a fuller knowledge of men and manners which contact with the bright minds in the profession ensures. My heart, or a good bit of it at least, has stayed with those who bestowed on me these treasures. Many a day I have felt it turn towards this city [Montreal] to the dear friends I left there, my college companions, my teachers, my old chums, the men with whom I lived in closest intimacy, and in parting from whom I felt the chordæ tendineæ [the tendons of the heart valves] grow tense.[56]

On another occasion he wrote of "the things that should accompany old age: fairly good health to the end, an unceasing interest in life, and the affectionate esteem of a large circle of friends." [57] As his career progressed, Osler took his many honors as signs of affection. He would say, "How my friends have pushed me forward!" [58]

The psychologist Daniel Levinson has pointed out that friendship among today's American males is remarkable largely for its absence.[59] Most men have wide circles of acquaintances based on shared activities but enjoy few if any intimate friendships. What can we learn from Osler's? He did not write weighty essays about friendship. However, three of the authors on his bedside reading list for medical students—Plutarch, Montaigne, and Emerson— wrote such essays, and their views merit summaries.

Plutarch's "How to Distinguish a Flatterer from a Friend" came in the context of a large body of literature on friendship in the classical world of Greece and Rome. Aristotle, for example, had classified friendship according to whether it was based on ulterior motives, pleasure, or mutual benefit. The happy, well-adjusted person should fill his or her life mainly with friendships of the latter type.[60] Plutarch was also heavily influenced by the Stoic philosophers, who held that only the wise and good person could be a friend. He suggested that flatterers find easy marks in persons suffused with self-love. Flatterers heap on praise and approval to enhance the intended victim's self-esteem, and they may feign similar interests and attitudes. Plutarch proposed that friends, unlike flatterers, are always willing to render sound advice that stings when first heard. As he put it, "a friend is like a musician, he loosens here and tightens there, and consequently, although he may often be likeable, he *always* does good." A second way to distinguish between friends and flatterers is that true friends are seldom possessive; rather, they share friends freely. Among Plutarch's other recommendations were (1) to suppress self-love and self-importance; (2) to praise before criticizing; (3) to pursue high goals; (4) to tolerate envy and criticism; and (5) above all, to be candid and sincere.[61]

Montaigne's essay "Of Friendship" dealt more with idealized or perfect friendship as reflected by his own four-year relationship with a slightly older man named Etienne de la Boetie. For Montaigne, "true friendship"—as distinguished from "common friendship" based on chance acquaintance and convenience—was a "noble relationship" that surpasses all else in life. The two souls are as one, each giving of himself "so wholly to his friend that he has nothing left to distribute elsewhere." He placed this type of male friendship on a much higher plane than his relationships with women, being "more active, more scorching, and more intense." True friends shared everything: "wills, thoughts, judgments, goods, wives, children, honor and life," the relationship being "that of one soul in two bodies." Montaigne never recovered from La Boetie's death, considering their relationship to have been the high point of his life.[62]

Emerson's "Friendship" suggests a more utilitarian position: "Friends such as we desire are dreams and fables." He did not crave a soulmate yet was "not so ungrateful as not to see the wise, the lovely, and the noble-minded as from time to time they pass my gate." The keys to friendship are sincerity and tenderness, neither of which comes easily. We are sincere to ourselves, but "at the entrance of a second person, hypocrisy begins." A friend is "a sort of paradox of nature" who allows mutual affirmation based on trust. Tenderness is difficult to describe in words, for "we can scarce believe that so much character can subsist in another as to draw us by love." Emerson differed with Plutarch in that he held self-love to be essential for friendship, but what he called self-love we would call healthy self-acceptance as opposed to narcissism:

"We must be our own, before we can be another's." We must also acknowledge the limits of friendship, for ultimately we are alone. Friendship is fraught with disappointments, but we must be brave enough to risk it. Emerson wrote, "The only reward of virtue is virtue: the only way to have a friend is to be one." [63]

Osler enjoyed a vast network of acquaintances and a few close friends drawn from different stages of his life. There were his boyhood friends, his medical friends, and a few friends at large. He does not seem to have sought perfect friendships, as Montaigne did. He chose instead to affirm others in a wide variety of settings and to allow them to affirm him in turn.[64] The historian Fielding H. Garrison wrote shortly after Osler's death that he

> had the gift of making almost any one feel for the moment as if he were set apart as a valued friend, and so became, in effect, a kind of universal friend to patients, pupils, and colleagues alike. But there was nothing of the politician in him. . . . Such an effective concentration of the "fluid, attaching character" has seldom been found in a single personality." [65]

This quality, perhaps more than anything else, explains his enormous popularity among contemporaries.

MAINTAIN OUTSIDE INTERESTS

Osler might be called a workaholic, and to some extent he was. However, he knew the pitfalls: "One cannot practise medicine alone and practise it early and late, as so many of us have to do, and hope to escape the malign influences of a routine life." [66] Medicine was by no means unique in this regard: "Professional work of any sort tends to narrow the mind, to limit the point of view and to put a hall-mark on a man of a most unmistakable kind." [67] Osler stressed to young physicians the importance of outside interests:

> Do not get too deeply absorbed [in your work] to the exclusion of all outside interests. Success in life depends as much upon the man as on the physician. Mix with your fellow students, mingle with their sports and their pleasures. . . . You are to be members of a polite as well as of a liberal profession and the more you see of life

outside the narrow circle of your work the better equipped will you be for the struggle.[68]

He was "constantly urging students to have a hobby" and suggested that they start early:[69]

> The young doctor should look about early for an avocation, a pastime, that will take him away from patients, pills, and potions. . . . No man is really happy or safe without one, and it makes precious little difference what the outside interest may be—botany, beetles or butterflies, roses, tulips, or irises, fishing, mountaineering or antiquities—anything will do so long as he straddles a hobby and rides it hard.[70]

Osler recognized that hobbies buffer us against the unexpected: "With a hobby a man is reasonably secure against the whips and arrows of the most outrageous fortune." [71]

Osler's main hobby was book collecting (see also Chapter 2). He loved everything about books. He collected first editions and aspired to owning all editions of a few books such as Sir Thomas Browne's *Religio Medici*. His enormous library included 104 incunabula (books published before the year 1501). He often spoke of "sanctifying his fee" for seeing patients by book purchases. He wrote, "Trite but true, is the comment of Seneca—'If you are fond of books you will escape the ennui of life, you will neither sigh for evening, disgusted with the occupations of the day—nor will you live dissatisfied with yourself or unprofitable to others.' " [72] He shared his books with friends and students, and nothing gave him more delight than finding a copy that filled a niche in someone else's library.

Osler loved books in part because they stood for culture, which he considered essential for physicians: "A physician may possess the science of Harvey and the art of Sydenham, and yet there may be lacking in him those finer qualities of heart and head which count for so much in life." [73] Moreover,

> On account of the intimate personal nature of his work, the medical man, perhaps more than any other man, needs that higher education of which Plato speaks,—"that education is virtue from youth upwards, which enables a man eagerly to pursue the ideal perfection." It is not for all, nor can all attain to it, but there is comfort and help in the pursuit, even though the end is never reached. . . . The all-important thing is to get a relish for the good company of the race in a

daily intercourse with some of the great minds of all ages. Now, in the spring-time of life, pick your intimates among them, and begin a systematic cultivation of their works. Many of you will need a strong leaven to raise you above the dough in which it will be your lot to labor.[74]

He urged young physicians to understand that love of books applies to any hobby:

> Every day do some reading or work apart from your profession. I fully realize, no one more so, how absorbing is the profession of medicine; how applicable to it is what Michelangelo says: "There are sciences which demand the whole of a man, without leaving the least portion of his spirit free for other distractions"; but you will be a better man and not a worse practitioner for an avocation. I care not what it may be; gardening or farming, literature or history or bibliography, any one of which will bring you into contact with books.[75]

Osler recognized that book collecting, like any hobby, expresses personality: "A library represents the mind of its collector, his fancies and foibles, his strength and weakness, his prejudices and preferences." Finally, he loved books because they provided another avenue toward a reference group, the people he wished to resemble. Thus, he wrote:

> It was the height of my ambition as a teacher to live up to the ideals of Morgan and Rush, of Hosack and Gerhard, of Bartlett and Drake, of Jackson and Bigelow. To know and to make known to students the lives and works of these men was a labour of love. Their works were collected and, what is more, read, and a regret remains that lack of time prevented the completion of many projected bio-bibliographic sketches.[76]

Osler's love of books was to a large extent the basis for his continued reputation as one of the most broadly informed physicians of all time. As one of his students mused, "Among general scholars he held his own so easily and with such charming grace that one often wondered how he found the time to keep abreast of medical progress." [77]

Although books became his obsession, Osler had many other interests. As was the style of professors in his day, he took extended summer vacations during which he often caught up with his reading and writing. Dr. Henry Barton Jacobs of Baltimore often went with him and recalled:

> It often seemed that in these vacations his thoughts were more keen and original than even in his days of work, but they were allowed to run into new channels with a spirit of boyishness and fun which captured the interest and admiration of all those around him. Then would appear those most truly characteristic traits of his nature, the love of his fellowmen, the love of service to others, and his un-bounding youthfulness of spirit. To these might be added the great reverence for the past with its heroes of contemplation and discov-ery, and great respect for the slowly moving yet beneficent laws of nature, often referred to by him as good old Doctor Time. The joy of living was ever uppermost in his mind coupled with the desire of giving joy to his companions.[78]

Osler liked sightseeing and went about it with "the enthusiasm of a boy," explaining to his companions "all the history of this or that object seen, constantly drawing upon his inexhaustible fund of knowledge, whether of literature, or local history, or of the hidden secrets of human nature." In London, for example, nothing "aroused his enthusiasm to a higher pitch, than [the] search for the great things in medical history which London afforded." In Cannes "he took the greatest pleasure in seeing the beauty of the place." [79] Although Osler had been good at competitive sports when young, he knew how to play without competing. As a friend recalled, "We had a game of croquet, he played very badly but took it lightheartedly as we all did." [80] On a vacation on the north coast of Cornwall, he observed that "the bathing [is] excellent & the golf links very good. I have put Revere into the hands of the Pro & we are now playing nine holes every afternoon. The fishing is very good, Isaac [Revere] says, but the fish do not bite!" [81] These comments make it clear that while Osler may indeed have been a workaholic to some extent, he knew the importance of play and was good at it.

ANSWER THE BIG QUESTIONS

Osler's chipper attitude and outgoing nature belied his taking seriously the "Big Questions" of our existence. Where do we come from? Is there a God? Is there an afterlife? Or, as Albert Einstein succinctly put it, is the universe ultimately a friendly place or not? The simple faith into which Osler was born was rocked by Charles Darwin's *Origin of the Species* (see Chapter 2). William Osler "saw Darwin once. . . . He was a most kindly old man, of large frame, with great bushy beard and eyebrows." [82] The more Osler thought about Darwinism, the more he took comfort in the promise of the emerging science. In 1894 he seemed to embrace what has been called social Darwinism without denying the possibility of a divine First Cause:

> In no way has biological science so widened the thoughts of men as in its application to social problems. That throughout the ages, in the gradual evolution of life, one unceasing purpose runs; that progress comes through unceasing competition, through unceasing selection and rejection; in a word, that evolution is the one great law controlling all living things, "the one divine event to which the whole creation moves," this conception has been the great gift of biology to the nineteenth century. [83]

He could even say that "Charles Darwin has so turned man right-about-face that, no longer looking back with regret upon a Paradise lost, he feels already within the gates of a Paradise regained." [84]

But if Osler found comfort in the new science, he found even greater comfort in the writings of his mentor, Sir Thomas Browne. Two centuries before Darwin, Browne struggled mightily with conflicts between Biblical religion and science. He wrote, "That Miracles are ceased, I can neither prove, nor absolutely deny; much less define the time and period of their cessation." [85] He began the *Religio Medici* with this famous passage:

> For my Religion, though there be several circumstances that might persuade the world I have none at all, as the general scandal of my profession, the natural course of my studies, the indifference of my behaviour, and discourse in matters of Religion, neither violently defending one, nor with that common ardor and contention opposing another; yet in despite hereof I dare, without usurpation, assume the honorable style of a Christian. [86]

Osler considered the *Religio Medici* to be "a *tour de force*, a daring attempt to combine scepticism with humble faith in the Christian religion." [87] Among Osler's frequent themes were the ephemeral nature of reputations and the fatuity of egotism. He lectured at

Yale that man "regards himself as the anthropocentric pivot around which revolve the eternal purposes of the Universe." Yet: "Knowing not whence he came, why he is here, or whither he is going, man feels himself of supreme importance, and certainly is of interest—to himself. Let us hope that he has indeed a potency and importance out of all proportion to his somatic insignificance." [88]

Osler's fascination with the metaphysical showed in what he called the "Death, Heaven and Hell" corner of his library at Oxford. He collected books about spiritualism, immortality, longevity, premature burial, preexistence, dreams, ghosts, witchcraft, euthanasia, embalming, cremation, resurrection, "self-murder," and related topics.[89] He was fascinated by near-death experiences. Here too he may have taken inspiration from Sir Thomas Browne, who wrote:

> It is observed that men sometimes upon the hour of their departure, do speak and reason above themselves. For then the soul begins to be freed from the ligaments of the body, begins to reason like herself, and to discourse in a strain above mortality.[90]

Browne talked about the various kinds of death:

> Now besides this literal and positive kind of death, there are others whereof Divines make mention, and those, I think, not merely Metaphorical, as Mortification, dying unto sin and the world; therefore, I say, every man has a double Horoscope, one of his humanity, his birth; another of his Christianity, his baptism . . . the way to be immortal is to die daily, nor can I think I have the true Theory of death.[91]

Browne preferred to dwell mainly on the positive alternative:

> I thank God, and with joy I mention it, I was never afraid of Hell, nor never grew pale at the description of that place; I have so fixed my contemplations on Heaven, that I have almost forgot the Idea of Hell, and I am afraid rather to lose the joys of the one than endure the misery of the other.[92]

Osler's chance to deliver his own views on science and immortality came in 1904, when he was asked to give the Ingersoll Lecture at Harvard. The will of a Miss Caroline Haskell Ingersoll of Keene, New Hampshire, had established the lectureship on the immortality of man from the perspective of either a clergyman or a layman. Osler accepted the invitation to give the sixth lecture in the

series at the urgings of his colleague William H. Welch and of
Harvard's president, Charles William Eliot. Osler began candidly:

> One of my colleagues, hearing that I was to give this lecture, said
> to me, "What do you know about immortality? You will say a few
> pleasant things, and quote the 'Religio Medici,' but there will be
> nothing certain." In truth, with his wonted felicity, my life-long
> mentor, Sir Thomas Browne, has put the problem very well when
> he said, "A dialogue between two infants in the womb concerning
> the state of this world might handsomely illustrate our ignorance of
> the next, whereof, I think, we yet discourse in Plato's den—the cave
> of transient shadows—and are but embryonic philosophers." Than
> the physician, no one has a better opportunity to study the attitude
> of mind of his fellow-men on the problem.

Osler proceeded to divide humans into three groups according to
their views on the afterlife. These were the Laodiceans, who, like
the lukewarm early Christians of Laodicea, professed belief but did
not allow it to influence their lives; the Gallioneans, who, like such
Roman officials as the aloof Junius Gallio, were unconcerned
about the issue of immortality; and the Teresians, who, like the
nuns and friars who followed St. Teresa, took religious faith as the
controlling force in their lives. Most people were Laodiceans:

> Practical indifference is the modern attitude of mind; we are
> Laodiceans,—neither hot nor cold, but lukewarm, as a very su-
> perficial observation will make plain. . . . Let us eat and drink; let
> us enjoy every hour saved from that eternal silence. . . . Even our
> more sober friends, as we see them day by day, interested in stocks
> and strikes, in base-ball and "bridge," arrange their view of this world
> entirely regardless of what may be beyond the flaming barriers—
> *flammantia mœnia mundi*. Where, among the educated and refined,
> much less among the masses, do we find any ardent desire for future
> life? It is not a subject of drawing-room conversation, and the man
> whose habit it is to button-hole his acquaintances and inquire ear-
> nestly after their souls, is shunned like the ancient Mariner.

Laodiceans were in truth "concerned less with the future life than
with the price of beef or coal."

The Gallionians, a smaller group, were agnostics whose lives
reflected indifference to the issue of afterlife:

> Like Gallio, they care for none of these things, and live wholly
> uninfluenced by a thought of the hereafter. They have either

reached the intellectual conviction that there is no hope in the grave, or the question remains open, as it did with Darwin, and the absorbing interests of other problems and the every-day calls of domestic life satisfy the mind.

Osler reviewed four aspects of the impact of science. First, the theory of evolution had weakened "the Sunday story from orthodox pulpits," and critical study of the Bible had weakened its claim of divine revelation. Second, "modern psychological science dispenses altogether with the soul." Third, science had been unable to identify spirits. And finally, modern science suggested that "the individual is nothing more than the transient off-shoot of a germ plasm."

Osler considered the most interesting group to be the true believers, or Teresians: "Though a little flock, this third group is the salt of the earth, so far as preserving for us a firm conviction of the existence of another and a better world." They were more likely to be women than men and nonscientists than scientists. Osler felt that religious belief is extremely useful and valid at least to the extent that it helps people:

> Though his philosophy finds nothing to support it, at least from the standpoint of Terence the scientific student should be ready to acknowledge the value of a belief in a hereafter as an asset to human life. In the presence of so many mysteries which have been unveiled, in the presence of so many yet unsolved, he cannot be dogmatic and deny the possibility of a future state. . . . He will recognize that amid the turbid ebb and flow of human misery, a belief in the resurrection of the dead and the life of the world to come is the rock of safety to which many of the noblest of his fellows have clung.

Osler acknowledged,

> The man of science is in a sad quandary to-day. He cannot but feel that the emotional side to which faith leans makes for all that is bright and joyous in life. Fed on the dry husks of facts, the human heart has a hidden want which science cannot supply.

He concluded with a statement that each person must work out his or her belief system:

> As perplexity of soul will be your lot and portion, accept the situation with a good grace. The hopes and fears which make us men

are inseparable, and this wine-press of Doubt each of you must tread alone. It is a trouble from which no man may deliver his brother or make agreement with another for him. . . . On the question before us wide and far your hearts will range from those early days. . . . In certain of you the changes and chances of the years ahead will reduce this to a vague sense of eternal continuity. . . . In a very few it will be begotten again as the lively hope of the Teresians; while a majority will retain the sabbatical interest of the Laoidicean. . . . Some of you will wander through all phases, to come at last, I trust, to the opinion of Cicero, who had rather be mistaken with Plato than be right with those who deny altogether the life after death; and this is my own *confessio fidei* [confession of faith].

Most of Osler's Ingersoll Lecture, including his division of humans into three groups according to their attitudes toward afterlife, was not original. He did, however, present some new data on dying. Between 1900 and 1904, he had studied 486 terminal patients at the Johns Hopkins Hospital "particularly with reference to the modes of death and the sensations of dying." He devised a questionnaire for the medical and nursing staff that included information about whether death was accompanied by bodily, mental, or spiritual distress. Of the 486 patients, according to the staff's findings,

> Ninety suffered bodily pain or distress of one sort or another, eleven showed mental apprehension, two positive terror, one expressed spiritual exaltation, one bitter remorse. The great majority gave no sign one way or the other; like their birth, their death was a sleep and a forgetting. The Preacher was right: in this matter man hath no preëminence over the beast,—"as the one dieth so dieth the other." [93]

Except for these brief observations about death scenes, President Eliot was deeply disappointed with the dearth of new information in Osler's lecture. Others, however, considered it to have been a brilliant exposition, and in one review of the entire Ingersoll series of lectures, it was commented that Osler's had "the most common-sense and was at the same time the most literary." [94]

In later years Osler was increasingly influenced by William James's philosophy of the pragmatic value of religious belief for many people.[95] He echoed James's *The Will to Believe* when he wrote, "We are at the mercy of our wills more than of our intellect in the formation of our beliefs, which we adopt in a lazy, haphazard way, without taking much trouble to inquire into their foundation." [96] Osler was consistent in his conviction that science and religion are not incompatible if one considers them separately. He told students:

> One and all of you will have to face the ordeal of every student in this generation who sooner or later tries to mix the waters of science with the oil of faith. You can have a great deal of both if you only keep them separate. The worry comes from the attempt at mixture.[97]

The extent to which Osler was comfortable with his own efforts to "have a great deal of both" is unclear. At Oxford he made a point of conducting ward rounds on Sunday mornings, a practice that one might interpret either way.[98] Visiting the Notre Dame in Paris, he reportedly dropped his coins in an offering marked "Prayers for those in Purgatory" with the explanation that he had "many friends there." [99] He never summarized his private religious views.[100] Although he is sometimes alleged to have been a radical humanist (that is, one who regards metaphysical phenomena of any kind as dangerous), his writings and sayings reflect an open mind. He held metaphysical beliefs to be dangerous only if, like medieval persons, "in seeking a heavenly home man lost his bearings on earth." He wrote,

> The greatest gift that nature or grace can bestow on a man is the *aequus animus*, the even-balanced soul; but unfortunately nature rather than grace, disposition rather than education, determines its existence. I cannot agree . . . that it is not to be acquired. On the contrary, I maintain that much may be done to cultivate a cheerful heart.[101]

Finally, he referred to "that remarkable saying of Prodicus (fifth century, B.C.), 'That which benefits human life is God.' " [102]

Osler felt strongly that faith can indeed benefit human life (see also Chapter 6). Lecturing in 1901 on the state of medicine, he declared that a

> noteworthy feature in modern treatment has been a return to psychical methods of cure, in which *faith in something is suggested* to the patient. After all, faith is the great lever of life. Without it, man can do nothing; with it, even with a fragment, as a grain of mustard-

seed, all things are possible to him. Faith in us, faith in our drugs and methods, is the great stock in trade of the profession. . . . In all ages the prayer of faith has healed the sick. . . . We enjoy, I say, no monopoly in the faith business. The faith with which we work, the faith, indeed, which is available to-day in everyday life, has its limitations. It will not raise the dead; it will not put in a new eye in place of a bad one . . . nor will it cure cancer or pneumonia, or knit a bone; but . . . such as we find it, faith is a most precious commodity, without which we should be very badly off.[103]

In 1910 he gave a lecture entitled "The Faith that Heals," in which he began,

Nothing in life is more wonderful than faith—the one great moving force which we can neither weigh in the balance nor test in the crucible. . . . To each one of the religions, past or present, faith has been the Jacob's ladder. Creeds pass; an inexhaustible supply of faith remains, with which man proceeds to rebuild temples, churches, chapels, and shrines.[104]

Someone who knew Osler throughout much of his adult life remarked, "No man ever led a more purely straightforward, spiritual life. In all his actions and in all his dealings the one ruling axiom throughout his life was the Golden Rule, and to it he consistently held in his relations with every man." [105] Osler, in summary, recognized the pragmatic usefulness of faith and addressed the "Big Questions" as best he could. And he also knew that the best strategy for dealing with the anxiety of ultimate fate is to live in day-tight compartments while serving others, for, as William James put it, "It is better to be than to define your being." [106]

BE COURAGEOUS

In his last major address, in 1919, Osler confided, "I have never succeeded in mastering philosophy—'cheerfulness was always breaking in.' " [107] But his medical practice gave frequent reminders of the inevitability of death or nonbeing, a reality heightened by his extensive experience at the autopsy table. He often stressed "the amount of damage which was often compatible with years of life and usefulness. The possibility of sufficient function to maintain life with extreme anatomical damage was often dwelt on and was a favorite subject." [108] At age 43, Osler told medical students that the best way to obtain peace of mind in one's later years is to live according to ideals that transcend self-interest:

> My message is chiefly to you, Students of Medicine, since with the ideals entertained now your future is indissolubly bound. The choice lies open, the paths are plain before you. Always seek your own interests, make of a high and sacred calling a sordid business, regard your fellow creatures as so many tools of the trade, and, if your heart's desire is for riches, they may be yours; but you will have bartered away the birthright of a noble heritage, traduced the physician's well-deserved title of the Friend of Man, and falsified the best traditions of an ancient and honourable Guild. On the other hand, I have tried to indicate some of the ideals which you may reasonably cherish. No matter though they are paradoxical in comparison with the ordinary conditions in which you work, they will have, if encouraged, an ennobling influence, even if only to say with Rabbi Ben Ezra, "what I aspired to be and was not, comforts me." And though this course does not necessarily bring position or renown, consistently followed it will at any rate give to your youth an exhilarating zeal and a cheerfulness which will enable you to surmount all obstacles—to your maturity a serene judgment of men and things, and that broad charity without which all else is nought—to your old age that greatest of blessings, peace of mind, a realization, maybe, of the prayer of Socrates for the beauty in the inward soul and for unity of the outer and the inner man; perhaps, of the promise of St. Bernard, "*pax sine crimine, pax sine turbine, pax sine rixa* [peace without crime, peace without turmoil, peace without quarrel]." [109]

Of the personal ideals Osler described in *Aequanimitas*, the third bears repeating: "to cultivate such a measure of equanimity as would enable me . . . to be ready when the day of sorrow and grief came to meet it with the courage befitting a man." [110]

Osler no doubt knew the literature on courage from Aristotle to Sir Thomas Browne but seldom discussed the subject per se. More immediately, he surely grew up with stories told by and about his father, Featherstone Lake Osler. As a young man in the seaport town of Falmouth, England, Featherstone Osler often flirted with disaster aboard ships. As a teenager, he was on the *Sappho* when it was nearly destroyed by Atlantic storms and was adrift for weeks. Later in the Royal Navy he was shipwrecked in the Barbados and survived only to be exposed to an epidemic of yellow fever. He served four more years in the Royal Navy before returning home, where he became a minister. Shortly after he married Ellen Pickton, he sailed from Falmouth to Quebec and was nearly shipwrecked on Egg Island in the Gulf of St. Lawrence. He went on to spend the next portion of his life as a missionary clergyman, living near the poverty level in a community that was six miles from the nearest blacksmith, twelve from the nearest post office, and fifteen from the nearest doctor.[111] It was perhaps Featherstone Osler's example that inspired four of the six Osler sons toward exceptional careers.[112] William Osler was not averse to taking on hazardous tasks that others might avoid, such as being in charge of the wards of a smallpox hospital.

Osler perceived that physicians, like clergy, should try to be strong as beacons to others. Those who knew him suspected that "when death touched him personally, though he suffered deeply he never permitted others to see within." [113] Osler told medical students,

> Often the best part of your work will have nothing to do with potions and powders, but with the exercise of an influence of the strong upon the weak, of the righteous upon the wicked, of the wise upon the foolish. To you, as the trusted family counsellor, the father will come with his anxieties, the mother with her hidden grief, the daughter with her trials, and the son with his follies. Fully one-third of the work you do will be entered in other books than yours. Courage and cheerfulness will not only carry you over the rough places of life, but will enable you to bring comfort and help to the weak-hearted and will console you in the sad hours when, like Uncle Toby [a character in *Tristram Shandy*, by Laurence Sterne], you have "to whistle that you may not weep." [114]

Osler knew that "the day of sorrow and grief" was inevitable:

> Sorrows and griefs are companions sure sooner or later to join us on our pilgrimage, and we have become perhaps more sensitive to them, and perhaps less amenable to the old time remedies of the physicians of the soul; but the pains and woes of the body, to which we doctors minister, are decreasing at an extraordinary rate, and in a way that makes one fairly gasp in hopeful anticipation.[115]

His own sorrow and grief were brought about by England's war with Germany. Lady Osler wrote, "Every morning we read of friends being mown down, all the youth and glory of the country, the young men we have known up here; and our only boy training in the park under our eyes—except that I can't look. Work is the only salvation. . . . W. O. is busy and trying to be cheerful." [116] He kept up a brave front.

Osler participated in the British war effort. Receiving a colonel's commission as a senior consultant to the English forces, he proudly wore his ill-fitting uniform and concerned himself with the numerous medical problems incident to war. A student noted that "Sir William worked like a Trojan . . . and helped in every way possible the advances in war medicine." [117] One colleague recalled that he was "charming, always interesting and interested; always giving in full measure of himself and of his time; always brave and smiling, and with an only son in France in the heavy artillery." [118] After Revere's death in 1917, he tried to work as though little or nothing had happened. A Philadelphia colleague wrote that Osler "taught us that to be brave when bravery seems impossible is true courage." [119] Finney, the Baltimore surgeon, similarly noted:

> His system of philosophy, which he had consistently preached and so faithfully practiced throughout a busy and fruitful life, had served him to the end. In the hour of triumph and success, it had helped him to bear with becoming humility all the honours that were heaped on him by an appreciative and admiring profession on both sides of the Atlantic. In the hour of trial, when grief-stricken and crushed to earth by the greatest of all sorrows that could have come to him, the untimely death in the World War of his only son, a youth of unusual promise, the pride and joy of his heart, he was still able with a supreme effort to manifest that "equanimity," about the virtues of which he had so eloquently discoursed in times gone by. Even "in the valley of the shadow of death," this quality of equanimity, and "the rod and the staff," with which he had been made familiar from his youth up, combined to comfort him.[120]

But silently, Osler suffered.Revere's death precipitated symptoms and signs of depression. Osler lost weight and he cried at night. It was in a weakened condition that on October 6, 1919, he developed a respiratory infection that evolved into pneumonia. The illness dragged on. Osler described his symptoms and signs objectively as though he were the physician rather than the patient.

There were grounds for optimism. However, as a colleague later revealed, an old Oxford janitor gave the correct prognosis:

> We who thought we knew him intimately were more sanguine than those further removed. Walking with [Charles Scott] Sherrington after the service, I heard from him the story of the old janitor at the physiological laboratory: "No, sir, I don't think Sir William will get better. You see, sir, it is like this: you know how Sir William, mostly on his way down to the hospital of a morning, would drop in for a few minutes to see you and the rest. Well, in the old days, coming in, and likewise going out, he had always a word for me. You know his style, sir, like giving a man a cheery dig in the ribs. But now these last months I have noticed him greeting you merry-like; but in between whiles his face has been grave as though he had something heavy on his mind, and he has walked in and out without once noticing me. It is Mr. Revere, sir, and Sir William won't get better." [121]

Osler faced his death with the same advice that he had given dying patients.[122] He attended to small details, kept up his correspondence, and made arrangements for the disposition of his beloved books. He wrote a friend of the possibility of an afterlife:

> No fever & pulse good; but the confounded thing drags on in an unpleasant way—and in one's 71st year the harbour is not far off. And such a happy voyage! & such dear companions all the way! And the future does not worry. It would be nice to find Isaac [Revere] there, with his friend Izaak Walton & others, but who knows.[123]

On the afternoon of December 29, 1919, Sir William Osler hemorrhaged into his chest cavity and died.

EPILOGUE

OSLER

ON

CHARACTER

Pursue Virtue Virtuously

Sir William Osler disliked lavish praise and
would probably have disapproved of the extent of his posthumous honors. Testimonials
were published, symposia held, societies
formed, lectureships established, hospital
wards and buildings named, medals struck,
busts sculpted, and portraits hung in far-
flung places, from the Royal College of Physicians in London to the town hall in Dundas,
Ontario. Even a Pullman railway car and a
Liberty ship were named after him.[1] His life
has been celebrated and dissected by at least
four full-length biographies and more than
1500 journal articles. How and why was he so
special to so many of his contemporaries, and
why does the adulation continue? Certainly,

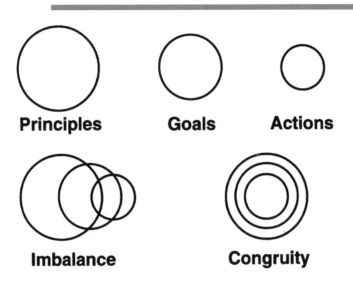

Character understood as congruity between benevolent principles, clear goals, and cheerfully-completed actions.

and by his own admission, he was not the platitudinous saint of our imaginations.

The same year that Osler published his textbook of medicine—1892—the Wistar Institute of Anatomy and Biology was formed in Philadelphia. At that time there was still some interest in phrenology, a now largely discredited branch of science given to correlating behavior with the external conformation of the cranium as an index to the weight and gyral patterns of the brain. Osler and other distinguished persons formed the Anthropologic Society and willed their brains to the Wistar Institute. Osler's brain was anatomically unremarkable.[2] Had Osler been asked what made him special, he would probably have pointed not to his own cranium but rather to the copy of Sir Thomas Browne's *Religio Medici* that he bought as a schoolboy, that guided him through adulthood, and that lay on his coffin as he rested in the Lady Chapel at Christ Church College on New Year's Day, 1920. Browne said, among other things: "Tread softly and circumspectly in this funambulous [tightrope-like] Track and narrow Path of Goodness: pursue Virtue virtuously." [3] It was from meticulous reading of Browne and other great authors of the past that Osler consciously cultivated what, for want of a better word, we call character.

What is character, and can it be taught? Osler, to reiterate, once quoted Plutarch to the effect that character is "long-standing habit." [4] The Victorian novelist Charles Reade said succinctly: "Sow an act, and you reap a habit. Sow a habit and you reap a character. Sow a character, and you reap a destiny." Osler might have defined character as doing one's best from hour to hour and from day to day as summed up by his philosophy of "day-tight compartments." We might elaborate that character is the essence of a life in which principles inform goals, goals inform actions, and actions are permeated with cheerfulness, energy, humility, and high sense of purpose. We might also insist that character requires love for fellow humans, love that was so well expressed by the deeds of that unpretentious man who wanted no other epitaph than that "I taught medical students in the wards."

Notes

FREQUENTLY CITED SOURCES

Frequently cited sources are listed here by author of original work, followed by full bibliographic citation; in the Notes, they are listed only by last name. William Osler is the author of all citations in the Notes unless otherwise stated. Full spellings of abbreviations for frequently cited medical and specialist journals are provided here for readers unfamiliar with citations of such literature; other journal names are spelled out in citations.

Abbreviations of Journals

Ann Intern Med: *Annals of Internal Medicine*
Arch Intern Med: *Archives of Internal Medicine*
BMJ: *British Medical Journal*

Bull Hist Med: *Bulletin of the History of Medicine*
CMAJ: *Canadian Medical Association Journal*
JAMA: *Journal of the American Medical Association*

Abbott, Maude E., ed.: Sir William Osler Memorial Number. *Bulletin No. IX of the International Association of Medical Museums and Journal of Technical Methods.* (Montreal, Canada: Privately printed, 1926).

Bacon, Sir Francis: *Essays* (Everyman's Library, London: J.M. Dent & Sons, 1992).

Barondess, Jeremiah A., McGovern, John P., and Roland, Charles G., eds.: *The Persisting Osler: Selected Transactions for the First Ten Years of the American Osler Society* (Baltimore: University Park Press, 1985).

Barondess, Jeremiah A., and Roland, Charles G., eds.: *The Persisting Osler—II: Selected Transactions of the American Osler Society, 1981–1900* (Malabar, Florida: Krieger, 1994).

Bean, William Bennett, ed.: *Sir William Osler: Aphorisms From His Bedside Teachings and Writings. Collected by Robert Bennett Bean, M.D. (1874-1944)* (New York: Henry Schuman, 1950).

Bett, W.R.: *Osler: The Man and the Legend* (London: William Heinemann, 1951).

Browne, Sir Thomas: *The Prose of Sir Thomas Browne.* Edited by Norman Endicott (New York: New York University Press, 1968).

Cushing, Harvey: *The Life of Sir William Osler* (Oxford: Clarendon Press, 1925).

Cervantes, Miguel de: *Don Quixote.* Translated by A. J. Close (New York: Alfred A. Knopf, 1991).

Emerson, Ralph Waldo: *Essays.* [and] *Essays: Second Series.* Introduction by Morse Peckham (Columbus, Ohio: Charles E. Merrill, 1969).

McGovern, John P. and Burns, Chester R., eds.: *Humanism in Medicine* (Springfield, Illinois: Charles C Thomas, 1973).

Montaigne, Michel de: *The Complete Works of Montaigne.* Translated by Donald M. Frame (Stanford, California: Stanford University Press, 1957).

Noble, Iris: *The Doctor Who Dared: William Osler* (New York: Julian Messner, 1959).

Osler, Sir William:

Aequanimitas. With other Addresses to Medical Students, Nurses, and Practitioners of Medicine. 3rd edition (Philadelphia: P. Blakiston's Son, 1932).

An Alabama Student. (London: Oxford University Press, 1908).

Men and Books. Collected and reprinted from *CMAJ* with an introduction by Earl F. Nation (Durham, North Carolina: Sacrum, 1987).

Selected Writings of Sir William Osler. Edited by G. L. Keynes (London: Oxford University Press, 1951).

The Evolution of Modern Medicine: A Series of Lectures Delivered at Yale University on the Silliman Foundation in April, 1913 (New Haven: Yale University Press, 1921).

Plutarch: *Essays.* Translated by Robin Waterfield (London: Penguin Books, 1992).

Pratt, Joseph H.: *A Year With Osler, 1886–1897: Notes taken at his Clinics in The Johns Hopkins Hospital* (Baltimore: The Johns Hopkins Press, 1949).

Reid, Edith Gittings: *The Great Physician: A Short Life of Sir William Osler* (London: Oxford University Press, 1931).

[Various contributors:] *Sir William Osler, Bart.: Brief Tributes to His Personality, Influence and Public Service* (Baltimore: Johns Hopkins Press, 1920).

[Various contributors:] *Oslerian Anniversary, Incorporating the Fitzpatrick Lecture for 1975.* (London: The Osler Club of London, 1976).

PREFACE

1. In several instances I relied heavily on Osler's recommended authors. These include Sir Thomas Browne on tolerance (Chapter 4) and skepticism (Chapter 5); Browne and

Cervantes on dealing with negative emotions (Chapter 4); Plutarch on listening (Chapter 7); and Plutarch, Montaigne, and Emerson on friendship (Chapter 8). Also, and as indicated in the text and notes, I have used works by Plutarch, Browne, and Emerson besides those specifically mentioned by Osler in the "Bed-Side Library for Medical Students" contained in the appendix to the *Aequanimitas* collection of addresses. One of my reasons for culling the collective wisdom of Osler's recommended authors is that with a few exceptions (most notably, the Bible and Shakespeare), most of these works are seldom read for pleasure today. Even Osler devotees have offered different lists. See, for example, Richard E. Verney, *The Student Life: The Philosophy of Sir William Osler* (Edinburgh and London: E. & S. Livingstone, 1957), 89–90; and Robert E. Rakel, "Modern Version of Osler's Bedside Library," in *Barondess and Roland*, 85–92.

2. For many years I have made extensive use of audiotapes obtained from the Nightingale-Conant Corporation (7300 North Lehigh Avenue, Niles, IL 60714).

3. "The Master-Word in Medicine," in *Aequanimitas*, 367.

4. Philip M. Teigen, "William Osler as Medical Hero," *Bull Hist Med* 1986 (60): 573–576.

5. H. P. Wright, "Osler—A Personal Tribute," *CMAJ* 1949 (61): 73–75.

CHAPTER 1

1. Fielding H. Garrison, *An Introduction to the History of Medicine*, 4th edition (Philadelphia: W. B. Saunders, 1929), 631.

2. "A Way of Life," in *Selected Writings*, 239.

3. See, for example, Dru Scott, *How to Put More Time in Your Life* (New York: Rawson, Wade, 1980); Charles R. Hobbs, *Time Power* (New York: Harper & Row, 1987); Stephen R. Covey, A. Roger Merrill, and Rebecca R. Merrill, *First Things First: To Live, to Love, to Learn, to Leave a Legacy* (New York: Simon & Schuster, 1994); and Stephanie Culp, *You Can Find More Time for Yourself Every Day* (Cincinnati: Betterway Books, 1994).

4. William DePrez Inlow, "The Medical Man as Philosopher: An Examination of the Pragmatism of William Osler," *Bull Hist Med* 1964 (38): 199–225.

5. Cushing, i, 20–31.

6. "After Twenty-Five Years," in *Aequanimitas*, 205.

7. John F. Fulton, "William Osler, The Humanist," *Arch Intern Med* 1949 (84): 149–158.

8. Cushing, i, 81.

9. "Teaching and Thinking," in *Aequanimitas*, 119.

10. "L'Envoi," in *Aequanimitas*, 450–451. See also "The Osler Dinner," *Medical News* [New York] 1905 (86): 854–860.

11. "Physic and Physicians as Depicted in Plato," in *Aequanimitas*, 53.

12. Browne, "Religio Medici," part 1, section 55, in *The Prose of Sir Thomas Browne*, 63. Here and elsewhere, I have taken the liberty to modernize Browne's spelling of certain words.

13. "Teacher and Student," in *Aequanimitas*, 37.

14. "Teaching and Thinking," in *Aequanimitas*, 124.

15. "Internal Medicine as a Vocation," in *Aequanimitas*, 141.

16. Ibid., 143.

17. Emerson, "Civilization," in *Society and Solitude* (Boston and New York: Houghton, Mifflin, 1904), 29–30.

18. "The Master-Word in Medicine," in *Aequanimitas*, 366–367.

19. "Teacher and Student," in *Aequanimitas*, 39.

20. "The Old Humanities and the New Science," in *Selected Writings*, 32.

21. Browne, "Christian Morals," part 1, section 1, in *The Prose of Sir Thomas Browne*, 371.

22. "Internal Medicine as a Vocation," in *Aequanimitas*, 138.

23. Cushing, i, 94.

24. Edmund J. A. Rogers, "Personal Reminiscences of the Earlier Years of Sir William Osler," in Abbott, 164.

25. "L'Envoi," in *Aequanimitas*, 449–450.

26. A. Schmidt, "Student Reminiscences, Montreal Period," in Abbott, 183.

27. "Books and Men," in *Aequanimitas*, 209.

28. Thomas McCrae, "The Influence of Pathology on the Clinical Medicine of William Osler," in Abbott, 39.

29. "Internal Medicine as a Vocation," in *Aequanimitas*, 145.

30. "Aequanimitas," in *Aequanimitas*, 7.

31. Cushing, i, 177.

32. "Teacher and Student," in *Aequanimitas*, 28.

33. "British Medicine in Greater Britain," in *Aequanimitas*, 170–171.

34. A. D. Blackader, "Osler's Early Work for Canadian Scientific Societies and as a Teacher in Montreal," in Abbott, 161.

35. "A Way of Life," in *Aequanimitas*, 240–241.

36. Ibid., 241.

37. Ibid., 242.

38. "The Army Surgeon," in *Aequanimitas*, 104.

39. "A Way of Life," in *Aequanimitas*, 249.

40. "The Master-Word in Medicine," in *Aequanimitas*, 361.

41. "After Twenty-Five Years," in *Aequanimitas*, 204.

42. Cushing, i, 631.

43. Ibid., 647.

44. W. W. Francis, R. H. Hill, and Archibald Malloch, eds., *Bibliotheca Osleriana: A Catalogue of Books Illustrating the History of Medicine and Science Collected, Arranged, and Annotated by Sir William Osler, Bt., and Bequeathed to McGill University* (Oxford: Clarendon Press, 1929), 315–316.

45. Scott, *How to Put More Time*, 3 (see note 3).

46. Henry M. Hurd, "The Personality of William Osler in Baltimore," in Abbott, 263.

47. Richard L. Golden, "Osler's Legacy: *The Principles and Practice of Medicine*," in *Barondess and Roland*, 47–59.

48. Reid, 85.

49. Edmund J. A. Rogers, "Personal Reminiscences of the Earlier Years of Sir William Osler," in Abbott, 167–168.

50. Lawrason Brown, "Reminiscence from Baltimore and Oxford Period," in Abbott, 442.

51. J. Herbert Darey, "Student Reminiscences, Montreal Period," in Abbott, 180.

52. William S. Thayer, "Osler," in Abbott, 288.

53. Marian Osborne, "Recollections of Sir William Osler," in Abbott, 174.

54. "Teacher and Student," in *Aequanimitas*, 34.

55. Browne, "Religio Medici," part 1, section 42, in *The Prose of Sir Thomas Browne*, 49.

56. "Teacher and Student," in *Aequanimitas*, 37.

57. Charles R. Hobbs, *Time Power*, 36 (see note 3).

58. "The Master-Word in Medicine," in *Aequanimitas*, 360.

59. "The Student Life," in *Aequanimitas*, 401.

60. *Introductory Lecture on the Opening of the Forty-Fifth Session of the Medical Faculty, McGill University, October 1st, 1877* (Montreal: Dawson Brothers, 1877), 11.

61. "The Army Surgeon," in *Aequanimitas*, 105.

62. "The Medical Library in Post-Graduate Work," *BMJ* 1909 (2): 925–928.

63. Cushing, i, 182.

64. "A Way of Life," in *Aequanimitas*, 238–239.

65. Ibid., 245–246.

66. Wilder Penfield, "A Medical Student's Memories of the Regius Professor," in Abbott, 387.

67. "Alfred Stillé," in *An Alabama Student*, 247.

68. Cushing, ii, 502.

69. Ibid., 31.

70. Norman Gwyn, "The Early Life of Sir William Osler," in Abbott, 109.

71. "Chauvinism in Medicine," in *Aequanimitas*, 265.

72. "Doctor and Nurse," in *Aequanimitas*, 17.

73. "The Student Life," in *Aequanimitas*, 401.

74. "After Twenty-Five Years," in *Aequanimitas*, 191.

75. Reid, 219.

76. Covey, Merrill, and Merrill, *First Things First* (see note 3).

77. William S. Thayer, "Osler," in Abbott, 290.

78. Cushing, i, 354–355.

79. George Dock, "Dr. Osler's Use of Time," *Arch Intern Med* 1949 (84): 51–53

80. Cushing, i, 289–290.

81. Marian Osborne, "Recollections of Sir William Osler," in Abbott, 173.

82. William S. Thayer, "Osler," in Abbott, 289.

83. Cushing, i, 286.

84. Charles P. Emerson, "Reminiscences of Sir William Osler," in Abbott, 301.

85. William S. Thayer, "Osler," in Abbott, 290.

86. William S. Thayer, "Osler, the Teacher," in *Sir William Osler, Bart.*, 53.

87. Thomas McCrae, "Osler and Patient," in *Sir William Osler, Bart.*, 62.

88. Wilburt C. Davison, "Sir William Osler: Reminiscences," *Arch Intern Med* 1949 (84): 110–128.

89. Cushing, i, 242–243.

90. Reid, 133.

91. Emerson, "Reminiscences of Sir William Osler," 301.

92. Ibid, 302.

93. Norman Gwyn, "The Early Life of Sir William Osler," in Abbott, 143.

94. Noble, 42–43.

95. Scott, *How to Put More Time*, 69 (see note 3).

96. "The Master-Word in Medicine," in *Aequanimitas*, 361–362.

97. William S. Thayer, "Osler," in Abbott, 287.

98. Ibid., 289.

99. Albert Vander Veer, "William Osler, M.D.: Personal Reminiscences," *Charlotte Medical Journal* 1920 (81): 137–139.

100. Cushing, ii, 613.

101. J.M.T. Finney, "A Personal Appreciation of Sir William Osler," in Abbott, 282.

102. J. C. Wilson, "Dr. Osler in Philadelphia, Teacher and Clinician," in Abbott, 246. The quoted scripture is from Proverbs 22:29.

103. Wilder Penfield, "Osler's Voice," in McGovern and Burns, 34–40.

CHAPTER 2

1. Joseph Campbell, *The Hero With a Thousand Faces*, 2nd edition (Princeton, N.J.: Princeton University Press, 1968), 245–251, 391.

2. Daniel J. Levinson, Charlotte N. Darrow, Edward B. Klein, Maria H. Levinson, and Braxton McKee, *The Seasons of a Man's Life* (New York: Alfred A. Knopf, 1978). The important issue of gender differences is beyond the scope of this brief discussion. See Daniel J. Levinson, and Judy D. Levinson, *The Seasons of a Woman's Life* (New York: Alfred A. Knopf, 1996).

3. "Doctor and Nurse, in *Aequanimitas*, 19.

4. Cushing, i, 53.

5. Browne, "Religio Medici," part 1, section 16, in *The Prose of Sir Thomas Browne*, 21.

6. "The Collecting of a Library," in *Selected Writings*, 255.

7. "The Master-Word in Medicine," in *Aequanimitas*, 359.

8. Cushing, i, 81.

9. Ibid., ii, 52.

10. Ibid., 411.

11. "Chauvinism in Medicine," in *Aequanimitas*, 267.

12. "Teacher and Student," in *Aequanimitas*, 32–33.

13. "Teaching and Thinking," in *Aequanimitas*, 122.

14. "Internal Medicine as a Vocation," in *Aequanimitas*, 133.

15. "The Army Surgeon," in *Aequanimitas*, 101.

16. "Letters to my House Physicians," in *Selected Writings*, 164–165.

17. "The Royal Medical Society of Edinburgh," *Scottish Medical and Surgical Journal* 1907 (20): 239–246.

18. "Nicolaus Steno," in *Men and Books*, 1.

19. "The Influence of Louis on American Medicine," in *An Alabama Student*, 210.

20. "Chauvinism in Medicine," in *Aequanimitas*, 273.

21. Ibid., 281–282.

22. "The Reserves of Life," *St. Mary's Hospital Gazette* 1907 (13): 95–98.

23. Reid, 153.

24. "Unity, Peace, and Concord," in *Aequanimitas*, 428–429.

25. "On the Educational Value of the Medical Society," in *Aequanimitas*, 334.

26. Cushing, ii, 225.

27. "Chauvinism in Medicine," in *Aequanimitas*, 280.

28. "On the Educational Value of the Medical Society," in *Aequanimitas*, 345. The quotation is adapted from Rudyard Kipling, "The Long Trail."

29. Browne, "Religio Medici," part 1, section 55, in *The Prose of Sir Thomas Browne*, 63.

30. "A Backwood Physiologist," in *An Alabama Student*, 185.

31. Cushing, ii, 262.

32. Ibid., 442.

33. Ibid., 494.

34. Bett, 4.

35. Edmund J. A. Rogers, "Personal Reminiscences of the Earlier Years of Sir William Osler," in Abbott, 164. See also Claus A. Pierach, "Was Osler *Verdeutsched?*" *Arch Intern Med* 1996 (156): 1502–1504.

36. "The Student Life," in *Aequanimitas*, 401–402.

37. Ibid., 406.

38. "Unity, Peace and Concord," in *Aequanimitas*, 429–430.

39. Ibid., 432.

40. "Chauvinism in Medicine," in *Aequanimitas*, 271.

41. "Internal Medicine as a Vocation," in *Aequanimitas*, 135. The quoted verse is probably traditional, after William Cowper's "The Progress of Error."

42. "Chauvinism in Medicine," in *Aequanimitas*, 267.

43. "British Medicine in Greater Britain," in *Aequanimitas*, 188.

44. Thomas R. Brown, "Osler and the Student," in *Sir William Osler, Bart.*, 57.

45. "Medicine in the Nineteenth Century," in *Aequanimitas*, 224.

46. "Specialism in the General Hospital," *Johns Hopkins Hospital Bulletin* 1913 (24): 167–171.

47. Reid, 119.

48. "The Leaven of Science," in *Aequanimitas*, 75.

49. William White, "The Biographical Essays of Sir William Osler and Their Relation to Medical History," *Bull Hist Med* 1939 (7): 28–48.

50. "Harvey and His Discovery," in *An Alabama Student*, 296.

51. *The Evolution of Modern Medicine*, 218.

52. "Israel and Medicine," in *Men and Books*, 60.

53. *The Evolution of Modern Medicine*, 10–11.

54. "British Medicine in Greater Britain," in *Aequanimitas*, 166.

55. "Physic and Physicians as Depicted in Plato," in *Aequanimitas*, 65.

56. "Chauvinism in Medicine," in *Aequanimitas*, 266.

57. "The Treatment of Disease," *Canada Lancet* 1909 (42): 899–912.

58. "Teaching and Thinking," in *Aequanimitas*, 121–122.

59. "Medicine in the Nineteenth Century," in *Aequanimitas*, 219–262.

60. J. A. Chatard, "Osler and the Book and Journal Club," in *Sir William Osler, Bart.*, 95.

61. "Chauvinism in Medicine," in *Aequanimitas*, 288.

62. "The Coming of Age of Internal Medicine in America," *International Clinics* 1915 (4): 1–5.

63. "Vienna After Thirty-Four Years," *JAMA* 1908 (50): 1523–1525.

64. Cushing, ii, 177.

65. A. D. Kelly, "Organization Man," *Canadian Journal of Surgery* 1970 (13): 335–340.

66. Cushing, i, 188.

67. Henry M. Hurd, "The Personality of William Osler in Baltimore," in Abbott, 262.

68. Thomas B. Futcher, "Influence on the Relation of Medicine in Canada and the United States," in *Sir William Osler, Bart.*, 69.

69. Henry M. Thomas, "Some Memories of the Development of the Medical School and of Osler's Advent," in *Sir William Osler, Bart.*, 16.

70. Louis Hamman, "Osler and the Tuberculosis Work of the Hospital," in *Sir William Osler, Bart.*, 65–66.

71. Cushing, ii, 49.

72. Henry M. Hurd, "Some Early Reminiscences of William Osler," in *Sir William Osler, Bart.*, 105.

73. A. M. Cook, "William Osler and the Royal College of Physicians of London," in *Oslerian Anniversary*, 6–7.

74. "The Functions of a State Faculty," *Maryland Medical Journal*, May 15, 1897 (37): 73–77.

75. Kelly, "Organization Man" (see note 65)

76. Lewellys F. Barker, "Osler as Chief of a Medical Clinic," in *Sir William Osler, Bart.*, 30–31.

77. "The Functions of a State Faculty" (see note 74).

78. "The Growth of a Profession," *Canada Medical and Surgical Journal* 1885–1886 (14): 129–155.

79. "The Army Surgeon," in *Aequanimitas*, 110.

80. "Chauvinism in Medicine," in *Aequanimitas*, 269.

81. "On the Educational Value of the Medical Society," in *Aequanimitas*, 335–336. The Coans were followers of the Hippocratic school at Cos, whereas the Cnidians were a rival school at Cnidus, a peninsula off the Ionian Coast; the humoralists were followers of Hippocrates' humoral theory of disease, whereas the solidists (from the first century B.C.) interpreted disease as a disordered arrangement of the atoms in the body; the Brunonians were followers of the heretical eighteenth-century Scottish physician John Brown, whereas the Broussaisians were followers of the French physician François-Joseph-Victor Broussais.

82. "Unity, Peace and Concord," in *Aequanimitas*, 438–439.

83. "On the Educational Value of the Medical Society," in *Aequanimitas*, 333.

84. Stephen R. Covey, A. Roger Merrill, and Rebecca R. Merrill, *First Things First: To Live, to Love, to Learn, to Leave a Legacy* (New York: Simon & Schuster, 1994), 44–74.

85. Marcia C. Noyes, "Osler's Influence on the Library of the Medical and Chirurgical Faculty of the State of Maryland," in *Sir William Osler, Bart.*, 98.

86. "The Leaven of Science," in *Aequanimitas*, 94.

87. "License to Practice," *JAMA* 1889 (12): 651–654.

88. Cushing, ii, 69–70.

89. Ibid., i, 344.
90. Ibid., ii, 43–44.
91. Ibid., 166–167.
92. "Books and Men," in *Aequanimitas*, 212.
93. "On the Library of a Medical School," *Johns Hopkins Hospital Bulletin* 1907 (18): 109–111.
94. W. W. Francis, "At Osler's Shrine," *Bulletin of the Medical Library Association* 1937 (26): 1–8. See also Charlotte Gray, "The Osler Library: A Collection That Represents the Mind of its Collector," *CMAJ* 1982 (119): 1442–1445.
95. "An Alabama Student," in *An Alabama Student*, 1–18. The quoted verse is adapted from Matthew Arnold, "Rugby Chapel."

CHAPTER 3

1. Cushing, i, 624.
2. "The Collecting of a Library," in *Selected Writings*, 254–255.
3. Cushing, i, 36.
4. Ibid., 36–37.
5. Wilder Penfield, "Osler's Voice," in McGovern and Burns, 34–40.
6. Cushing, i, 50.
7. "Canadian Fresh-water Polyzoa," *Canadian Naturalist* 1883 (10[n.s.]): 399–406.
8. Cushing, i, 48
9. Ibid., 57.
10. Ibid., 62.
11. Ibid., 67.
12. Ibid., 95.
13. "The Master-Word in Medicine," in *Aequanimitas*, 353.
14. Ibid., 355.
15. Cushing, i, 83.
16. "The Collecting of a Library," in *Selected Writings*, 258.
17. Noble, 39–40.
18. Ibid.
19. "The Student Life," in *Aequanimitas*, 420–421.
20. Bean, 87.
21. Reid, 54.
22. Cushing, i, 121.
23. Ibid., 245.
24. "Sir Thomas Browne," in *An Alabama Student*, 276–277.
25. Cushing, ii, 24–25.
26. Ibid., 660.
27. Ibid., 509.
28. "Physic and Physicians as Depicted in Plato," in *Aequanimitas*, 47.
29. R. Palmer Howard, "The Men Who Inspired Osler," in McGovern and Burns, 41–48. See also Benjamin Spector, "Osler: An Exemplar of Litterae, Scientia, Praxis, and Doctrina," *Bull Hist Med* 1949 (23): 378–386.
30. *Thomas Linacre* (Cambridge: Cambridge University Press, 1908), 6–7.
31. "British Medicine in Greater Britain," in *Aequanimitas*, 167–168.
32. "Harvey and his Discovery," in *An Alabama Student*, 333–334.
33. Cushing, ii, 64.
34. *The Evolution of Modern Medicine*, 190.
35. Ibid.
36. "The Evolution of Internal Medicine," in William Osler and Thomas McCrae, eds., *Modern Medicine: Its Theory and Practice* (Philadelphia: Lea Brothers, 1907), i, xxi.
37. "British Medicine in Greater Britain," in *Aequanimitas*, 174.

38. Ibid., 188.

39. Cushing, i, 513–514.

40. Ibid., 510.

41. Ibid., 404.

42. "William Pepper," in *An Alabama Student*, 231. The quoted verse is from Robert Louis Stevenson, "Underwoods."

43. "British Medicine in Greater Britain," in *Aequanimitas*, 169.

44. Linda Phillips-Jones, *Mentors & Protégés* (New York: Arbor House, 1982), 74–75.

45. Joseph H. Pratt, "Osler as His Students Knew Him," *Boston Medical and Surgical Journal* 1920 (182): 338–341.

46. Daniel J. Levinson, Charlotte N. Darrow, Edward B. Klein, Maria H. Levinson, and Braxton McKee, *The Seasons of a Man's Life* (New York: Alfred A. Knopf, 1978), 252–256. See also Daniel J. Levinson and Judy D. Levinson, *The Seasons of a Woman's Life* (New York: Alfred A. Knopf, 1996), 342–344.

47. Charles G. Roland, "Introduction—William Osler, 1849–1919, Commemorative Issue," *JAMA* 1969 (210): 2213.

48. Cushing, i, 404–405.

49. Ibid., 445.

50. "The Student Life," in *Aequanimitas*, 397.

51. "The Importance of Post-Graduate Study," *Lancet* 1900 (2): 73–75.

52. Cushing, ii, 123.

53. William S. Thayer, "Osler, The Teacher," in *Sir William Osler, Bart.*, 53.

54. "The Growth of a Profession," *Canada Medical and Surgical Journal* 1885–1886 (14): 129–155.

55. Cushing, ii, 76. The extent of Osler's qualms about coeducation is unclear. William H. Welch wrote that Osler was among those who were less than enthusiastic about the admission of women to Johns Hopkins on the same basis as men and that Osler did not sign a petition urging the university's Board of Trustees to accept the terms of a Women's Fund Committee that had raised funds enabling the medical school to open with the stipulation of equal opportunity for both sexes (Cushing, i, 387). However, the record is clear that Osler—whatever his qualms may have been—signed the petition. Alan M. Chesney wrote: "One is forced to the conclusion that Dr. Welch's memory must have played him false in this instance for at no place in the official record covering this particular period is there any intimation that the question of admitting women on the same terms as men was under discussion." See Chesney, *The Johns Hopkins Hospital and The Johns Hopkins University School of Medicine: A Chronicle* (Baltimore: Johns Hopkins Press, 1943), i, 193–219. The extent to which Osler's memory was cherished by such women physicians as Maude E. Abbott and Esther Rosencrantz suggests that he was at least as progressive as most men of his day on this issue.

56. "The Student Life," in *Aequanimitas*, 399–400.

57. C. N. B. Camac, ed., *Counsels and Ideals from the Writings of William Osler* (Boston: Houghton, Mifflin, 1905). For details on the Osler-Camac relationship, see Earl F. Nation, "The Influence of Osler on His Students: The Osler-Camac Correspondence Concerning *Counsels and Ideals from the Writings of William Osler*," *JAMA* 1969 (210): 2226–2231; and Earl F. Nation and John P. McGovern, eds., *Student and Chief: The Osler-Camac Correspondence* (Pasadena, Cal.: Castle, 1980).

58. Cushing, ii, 686.

59. "L' Envoi," in *Aequanimitas*, 447.

60. Ibid., 449.

61. "Unity, Peace and Concord," in *Aequanimitas*, 427.

62. Wilburt C. Davison, "Sir William Osler: Reminiscences," *Arch Intern Med* 1949 (84): 110–128.

63. "The Growth of a Profession," *Canada Medical and Surgical Journal*, 1885–1886 (14): 129–155.

64. Reid, 127.

65. Cushing, ii, 12.

66. Ibid., i, 417–418.

67. For a concise review, see Ann D. Carden, "Mentoring and Adult Career Development," *Consulting Psychologist* 1990 (18): 275–299. See also Laurent A. Daloz, *Effective Teaching and Mentoring* (San Francisco: Jossey-Bass, 1986).

68. Levinson et al., *The Seasons of a Man's Life*, 99–101 (see note 47).

69. Reid, 51.

70. Norman B. Gwyn, "The Letters of a Devoted Father to an Unresponsive Son," *Bull Hist Med* 1939 (7): 335–351. Johnson's criticism may have reflected, in part, displaced hostility actually meant for William Osler's father, the Reverend Featherstone Lake Osler, who had been a member of a committee appointed to investigate Johnson's activities at Weston.

71. "The Collecting of a Library," in *Selected Writings*, 257.

72. "The Master-Word in Medicine," in *Aequanimitas*, 353.

73. Cushing, i, 97.

74. See Jeremiah A. Barondess, "Cushing and Osler: The Evolution of a Friendship," in Barondess and Roland, 95–120; Barondess, "A Brief History of Mentoring," *Transactions of the American Clinical and Climatological Association* 1994 (106): 1–24; and John F. Fulton, *Harvey Cushing: A Biography* (Springfield, Ill.: Charles C Thomas, 1946).

75. "The Student Life," in *Aequanimitas*, 421–422.

76. Cushing, i, 377.

CHAPTER 4

1. Sir George Pickering, "Osler: Regius Professor of Medicine, Oxford," *JAMA* 1969 (210): 2268.

2. Browne, "Christian Morals", part 3, section 9, in *The Prose of Sir Thomas Browne*, 407.

3. Emerson, "Spiritual Laws," in *Essays*, 117.

4. "The Student Life," in *Aequanimitas*, 423.

5. "The Master-Word in Medicine," in *Aequanimitas*, 368.

6. "Aequanimitas," in *Aequanimitas*, 8. The quoted verse is from Robert Browning, "Rabbi Ben Ezra."

7. "Doctor and Nurse," in *Aequanimitas*, 15–16.

8. René Dubos, "The Despairing Optimist," *American Scholar* 1976 (Winter) (46): 10–18.

9. "The Treatment of Disease," *Canada Lancet* 1909 (42): 899–912.

10. "Teaching and Thinking: The Two Functions of a Medical School," in *Aequanimitas*, 117–118.

11. Reid, 23.

12. Emerson, "Worship," in *The Conduct of Life* (Boston: Ticknor and Fields, 1860), 191–192.

13. "The Master-Word in Medicine," in *Aequanimitas*, 368.

14. Ibid., 369.

15. "Unity, Peace, and Concord," in *Aequanimitas*, 442.

16. Bean, 86.

17. "Aequanimitas," in *Aequanimitas*, 8.

18. Cushing, i, 18.

19. Browne, "Religio Medici," part 2, section 13, in *The Prose of Sir Thomas Browne*, 87.

20. "Sir Thomas Browne," in *An Alabama Student*, 258.

21. Cushing, i, 132.

22. Reid, 55–56.

23. Cushing, ii, 636.

24. John F. Fulton, "William Osler, The Humanist," *Arch Intern Med* 1949 (84): 149–158.

25. Sir Geoffrey Keynes, "The Oslerian Tradition," *BMJ* 1968 (4): 599–604.

26. "The Inner History of the Johns Hopkins Hospital" (edited, annotated, and introduced by Donald G. Bates and Edward H. Bensley), *Johns Hopkins Medical Journal* 1969 (125): 184–194.

27. "The Functions of a State Faculty," *Maryland Medical Journal*, May 15, 1897 (37): 73–77.

28. Cushing, i, 543.

29. Ibid., ii, 36.

30. John Brett Langstaff, "Youthful Recollections," *JAMA* 1969 (210):2233–2235.

31. Cushing, i, 146.

32. Ibid, 228.

33. "The Student Life," in *Aequanimitas*, 397.

34. "The Master-Word in Medicine," in *Aequanimitas*, 356–358.

35. "A Way of Life," in *Selected Writings*, 247. The quoted verse is from George Herbert, "The Elixir." The literary allusion is to Bunyan's *Pilgrim's Progress*.

36. "Teacher and Student," in *Aequanimitas*, 33.

37. Cushing, i, 264.

38. Emile Holman, "Sir William Osler: Teacher and Bibliophile," *JAMA* 1969 (210): 2223–2225.

39. "Richard Lea MacDonnell," *New York Medical Journal*, 1891 (54):162.

40. "The Army Surgeon," in *Aequanimitas*, 103.

41. Reid, 220.

42. Cushing, ii, 206–207.

43. Ibid., i, 53.

44. "Obituary: Samuel W. Gross, M.D.," *Medical News* [Philadelphia] 1889 (54):474–476.

45. Browne, "Christian Morals," part 3, section 22, in *The Prose of Sir Thomas Browne*, 417.

46. Cushing, i, 220.

47. "L'Envoi," in *Aequanimitas*, 448.

48. Henry M. Thomas, "Some Memories of the Development of the Medical School and of Osler's Advent," in *Sir William Osler, Bart.*, 14.

49. Cushing, i, 649.

50. Howard A. Kelly, "Osler As I Knew Him in Philadelphia and in the Hopkins," in Abbott, 261.

51. Holman, "Sir William Osler: Teacher and Bibliophile" (see note 38).

52. Joseph H. Pratt, "Osler as his Students Knew Him," *Boston Medical and Surgical Journal* 1920 (182): 338–341.

53. Jeremiah A. Barondess, "A Hitherto Unpublished Appreciation of Sir William Osler by Doctor A. G. Gibson," *Johns Hopkins Medical Journal* 1977 (140): 47–55.

54. Browne, "Religio Medici," part 2, section 4, in *The Prose of Sir Thomas Browne*, 73.

55. Browne, "Christian Morals," part 1, section 28, in *The Prose of Sir Thomas Browne*, 383.

56. Browne, "Religio Medici," part 1, in *The Prose of Sir Thomas Browne*, section 6, 11.

57. Ibid., part 2, section 1, 66.

58. "Aequanimitas," in *Aequanimitas*, 6.

59. Ibid.

60. Joseph H. Pratt, "The Influence of Osler on the Practice of Medicine," *Boston Medical and Surgical Journal* 1927 (196): 83–89.

61. "Teacher and Student," in *Aequanimitas*, 39.

62. Cushing, i, 74.

63. Ibid., ii, 15.

64. "The Treatment of Disease," *Canada Lancet* 1909 (42): 899–912.

65. "John Locke as a Physician," in *An Alabama Student*, 68.

66. Ibid., 72.

67. Ibid., 107.

68. George E. Vaillant, *Adaptation to Life: How the Best and the Brightest Came of Age* (Boston: Little, Brown, 1977), 368.

69. "Teaching and Thinking," in *Aequanimitas*, 128.

70. "Robert Burton: The Man, His Book, His Library," in *Selected Writings*, 65.

71. Cushing, ii, 22–23.

72. Browne, "Christian Morals," part 1, section 15, in *The Prose of Sir Thomas Browne*, 376.

73. Ibid., part 3, section 12, 409.

74. Cervantes, *Don Quixote,* part 2, book 5, chapter 8, 60.

75. "Aequanimitas," in *Aequanimitas*, 7–8.

76. Reid, 74.

77. Edward B. Krumbhaar, "Additional Notes on Osler in Philadelphia," *Arch Intern Med* 1949 (84): 26–33.

78. "Professor Wesley Mills," *CMAJ* 1915 (5): 338–341.

79. Cushing, ii, 614–615.

CHAPTER 5

1. "The Leaven of Science," in *Aequanimitas*, 95.

2. "The Master-Word in Medicine," in *Aequanimitas*, 362.

3. "Teaching and Thinking," in *Aequanimitas*, 121.

4. "The Importance of Post-Graduate Study," *Lancet* 1900 (2): 73–75.

5. Wilburt C. Davison, "Sir William Osler: Reminiscences," *Arch Intern Med* 1949 (84): 110–128.

6. "Aequanimitas," in *Aequanimitas*, 9.

7. "Teaching and Thinking," in *Aequanimitas*, 120.

8. Cushing, ii, 245–246.

9. "Teaching and Thinking," in *Aequanimitas*, 128.

10. "Teacher and Student," in *Aequanimitas*, 29–30.

11. "Teaching and Thinking," in *Aequanimitas*, 128.

12. "Teacher and Student," in *Aequanimitas*, 26.

13. "Chauvinism in Medicine," in *Aequanimitas*, 279.

14. "The Master-Word in Medicine," in *Aequanimitas*, 349.

15. "On the Library of a Medical School," *Johns Hopkins Hospital Bulletin* 1907 (18): 109–111.

16. "Books and Men," in *Aequanimitas*, 210–211.

17. Cushing, ii, 81.

18. Ibid., 89.

19. *The Evolution of Modern Medicine*, 65.

20. "The Pathological Institute of a General Hospital," *Glasgow Medical Journal* 1911 (76): 321–333.

21. "On the Need of a Radical Reform in Our Methods of Teaching Senior Students," *Medical News* [New York] 1903 (82): 49–53.

22. "The Hospital as a College," in *Aequanimitas*, 315–316.

23. "The Army Surgeon," in *Aequanimitas*, 104.

24. "John Locke as a Physician," in *An Alabama Student*, 78.

25. Ibid., 101.

26. "The Influence of Louis on American Medicine," in *An Alabama Student*, 191.

27. Beth M. Belkin and Francis A. Neelon, "The Art of Observation: William Osler and the Method of Zadig," *Ann Intern Med* 1992 (116): 863–866.

28. "The Army Surgeon," in *Aequanimitas*, 105–106.

29. Thomas B. Futcher, "The Importance of Bed-side Study and Teaching," *CMAJ* 1935 (32): 357–364.

30. William G. MacCallum, "Osler as a Pathologist," in *Sir William Osler, Bart.*, 45–49.

31. "The Natural Method of Teaching the Subject of Medicine," *JAMA* 1901 (36): 1673–1679.

32. Lawrence J. Rhea, "Osler and Pathology," in Abbott, 13.

33. "The Natural Method of Teaching the Subject of Medicine" (see note 31).

34. "The Student Life," in *Aequanimitas* 411–412.

35. Warfield T. Longcope, "Random Recollections of William Osler, 1899–1918," *Arch Intern Med* 1949 (84): 93–103.

36. Cushing, i, 186.

37. "The Army Surgeon," in *Aequanimitas*, 109.

38. "The Student Life," in *Aequanimitas*, 405–406.

39. William B. Bean, "Nail Growth: 30 Years of Observation," *Arch Intern Med* 1974 (134): 497–502.

40. William S. Thayer, "Osler, The Teacher," in *Sir William Osler, Bart.*, 51–52.

41. "The Natural Method of Teaching the Subject of Medicine" (see note 31).

42. "Chauvinism in Medicine," in *Aequanimitas*, 281. The allusion to Homer probably refers to the *Iliad* (XI.514): "A leech [physician] is of the worth of many other men for the cutting out of arrows and the spreading of soothing simples."

43. Ibid., 289.

44. "An Introductory Address on Examinations, Examiners, and Examinees," *Lancet* 1913 (2): 1047–1050.

45. "The Treatment of Disease," *Canada Lancet* 1909 (42): 899–912.

46. "Teaching and Thinking," 124.

47. "The Student Life," in *Aequanimitas*, 405.

48. Ibid., 417.

49. "The Hospital as a College," in *Aequanimitas*, 313.

50. "What the Public Can Do in the Fight Against Tuberculosis" (Oxford: Privately printed for the Tuberculosis Exhibition & Conferences, Oxford, Nov. 8–13, 1909).

51. "The Student Life," in *Aequanimitas*, 412–413. The quoted verses are from William Cowper, "Winter Walk at Noon," and Alfred, Lord Tennyson, "Locksley Hall."

52. George T. Harrell, "Osler's Practice," in Barondess, McGovern, and Roland, 105–129.

53. "The Coming of Age in Internal Medicine in America," *International Clinics* 1915 (4): 1–5.

54. Davison, "Memories of Sir William Osler," *JAMA* 1969 (210): 2219–2222.

55. "After Twenty-Five Years," in *Aequanimitas*, 195.

56. "Teacher and Student," in *Aequanimitas*, 38–39.

57. *Lectures on the Diagnosis of Abdominal Tumors* (New York: D. Appleton, 1898), 191–192.

58. James B. Herrick, "William Osler: A Personal Note," *Arch Intern Med* 1949 (84): 46–50.

59. Browne, "Religio Medici," part 2, section 8, in *The Prose of Sir Thomas Browne*, 79.

60. Browne, "Pseudodoxia Epidemica," introduction, in *The Prose of Sir Thomas Browne*, 99.

61. Ibid., book 1, chapter 5, 118.

62. Browne, "Religio Medici," part 1, section 6, in *The Prose of Sir Thomas Browne*, 11.

63. Browne, "Pseudodoxia Epidemica," book 1, chapter 6, in *The Prose of Sir Thomas Browne*, 122.

64. "Elisha Bartlett, A Rhode Island Philosopher," in *An Alabama Student*, 112.

65. William G. MacCallum, "Osler as a Pathologist," in *Sir William Osler, Bart.*, 46.

66. "Chauvinism in Medicine," in *Aequanimitas*, 284.

67. Cushing, i, 594.

68. "The Leaven of Science," in *Aequanimitas*, 84.

69. "The Student Life," in *Aequanimitas*, 397–398.

70. Cushing, i, 593.

71. "On the Educational Value of the Medical Society," in *Aequanimitas*, 331–332.

72. Cushing, i, 594.

73. See Stephen D. Brookfield, *Developing Critical Thinkers: Challenging Adults to Explore Alternative Ways of Thinking and Acting* (San Francisco: Jossey-Bass, 1987).

74. "Aequanimitas," in *Aequanimitas*, 6–7.

75. "On the Educational Value of the Medical Society," 332–333.

76. Ilza Veith, "Sir William Osler, Acupuncturist," in Barondess, McGovern, and Roland, 125–129.

77. "Medicine in the Nineteenth Century," in *Aequanimitas*, 255.

78. "The Treatment of Disease" (see note 45).

79. Harry Toulmin, "Recollections, Johns Hopkins Period," in Abbott, 230.

80. Pratt, 63.

81. "The Student Life," in *Aequanimitas*, 419.

82. "Looking Back—1889," in *Men and Books*, 62.

83. Alan M. Chesney, *The Johns Hopkins Hospital and The Johns Hopkins University School of Medicine. A Chronicle* (Baltimore: Johns Hopkins Press, 1943), i, 312.

84. Cushing, i, 388.

85. Thomas R. Brown, "Osler and the Student," in *Sir William Osler, Bart.*, 55–56.

86. Henry M. Thomas, "Some Memories of the Development of the Medical School and of Osler's Advent," in *Sir William Osler, Bart.*, 16.

87. Reid, 46.

88. "The Medical Library in Post-Graduate Work," *BMJ* 1909 (2): 925–928.

89. "Teacher and Student," in *Aequanimitas*, 32.

90. Cushing, i, 321.

91. "The Medical Library in Post-Graduate Work" (see note 88).

92. William White, "*Æquanimitas*: Osler's Inspirational Essays," *Bull Hist Med* 1938 (6): 820–833.

93. "The Student-Life," in *Aequanimitas*, 400.

94. Cushing, i, 167.

95. "After Twenty-Five Years," in *Aequanimitas*, 201–202.

96. Reid, 147.

97. Neil McIntyre, "Osler and Medical Education," in *Oslerian Anniversary*, 16–23.

98. R. Palmer Howard, "William Osler: A 'Potent Ferment' at McGill," *Arch Intern Med* 1949 (84): 12–15.

99. Oliver Wendell Holmes, *Medical Essays, 1842–1882* (Boston: Houghton, Mifflin, 1883), 273–274.

100. "Looking Back—1889," in *Men and Books*, 62.

101. Cushing, i, 596.

102. Michael L. Friedland, "Oslerian Basis of Education in the Ambulatory Setting," *Academic Medicine* 1995 (70): 344–345.

103. "After Twenty-Five Years," in *Aequanimitas*, 200.

104. "Examinations, Examiners, and Examinees" (see note 44).

105. "The Natural Method of Teaching the Subject of Medicine" (see note 31).

106. Davison, "Sir William Osler: Reminiscences" (see note 5).

107. Cushing, i, 209.

108. "The Pathological Institute of a General Hospital" (see note 20).

109. Cushing, ii, 220.

110. *The Evolution of Modern Medicine*, 199.

111. "British Medicine in Greater Britain," in *Aequanimitas*, 181.

112. "The Influence of Louis on American Medicine," in *An Alabama Student*, 193.

113. *The Evolution of Modern Medicine*, 215.

114. "The Leaven of Science," in *Aequanimitas*, 92–93. Osler attributed the quotation to Hermann von Helmholtz.

115. "The Reserves of Life," *St. Mary's Hospital Gazette* 1907 (13): 95–98.

116. "The Leaven of Science," in *Aequanimitas*, 92.

117. "Teaching and Thinking," in *Aequanimitas*, 128.

118. "The Historical Development and Relative Value of Laboratory and Clinical Methods in Diagnosis: The Evolution of the Idea of Experiment in Medicine," in *Transactions of the Congress of American Physicians and Surgeons, Seventh Triennial Session* (New Haven, Conn.: By the Congress, 1907), 1–8.

CHAPTER 6

1. Arthur S. Freese, "He Was Family Doctor to the World," *Today's Health* 1968 (June): 39–41.

2. "The Old Humanities and the New Science," in *Selected Writings*, 33.

3. Gerald Weissmann, "Against Aequanimitas," *Hospital Practice* 1984 (June): 159–169.

4. With respect to such issues as managed care, a frequent question is "What would Osler do were he alive today?" In truth he had relatively little to say about the economic structure of medical practice. See, however, "The Future of the Medical Profession Under a Ministry of National Health," *Lancet* 1918 (1): 804–806.

5. Pratt, 79, 125, 173.

6. Wilder Penfield, "Hero Worship," *Arch Intern Med* 1949 (84): 104–109.

7. Cushing, i, 135–137.

8. Earl F. Nation, "Sir William Osler, the Master of Ewelme," *CMAJ* 1973 (109): 1128–1132.

9. Raymond D. Pruitt, "Dr. William and Dr. Will: A Study of Contrast in Greatness," in Barondess, McGovern, and Roland, 235.

10. James E. Paullin, "My First Medical Clinic with Dr. Osler," *Arch Intern Med* 1949 (84): 84–85.

11. *The Evolution of Modern Medicine*, 6–7. The quoted verse is from William Wordsworth, "Intimations of Immortality from Recollections of Early Childhood. An Ode," and the Latin phrase is from Lucretius, *De Rerum Natura*.

12. "On the Educational Value of the Medical Society," in *Aequanimitas*, 333.

13. "Chauvinism in Medicine," in *Aequanimitas*, 268.

14. Charles P. Emerson, "Reminiscences of Sir William Osler," in Abbott, 300.

15. "Teaching and Thinking," in *Aequanimitas*, 126.

16. "Nurse and Patient," in *Aequanimitas*, 149–159.

17. Marian Osborne, "Recollections of Sir William Osler," in Abbott, 173.

18. "The Student Life," in *Aequanimitas*, 404–405.

19. A. D. Gardner, "Some Recollections of Sir William Osler at Oxford," *JAMA* 1969 (210): 2265–2267.

20. Cushing, ii, 181–182.

21. The point has been made that in his psychotherapy Osler was influenced by the writings of Robert Burton. See Stanley W. Jackson, "Robert Burton and Psychological Healing," *Journal of the History of Medicine and Allied Sciences* 1989 (44): 160–178.

22. Thomas R. Brown, "Osler and the Student," in *Sir William Osler, Bart.*, 56.

23. Thomas McCrae, "Osler and Patient," in *Sir William Osler, Bart.*, 59.

24. Lewellys F. Barker, "Sir William Osler," *Evening Sun* [Baltimore], December 30, 1919.

25. Jeremiah A. Barondess, "A Hitherto Unpublished Appreciation of Sir William Osler by Doctor A. G. Gibson," *Johns Hopkins Medical Journal* 1977 (140): 47–55.

26. Cushing, i, 264.

27. Ibid., 161–162.

28. "Robert Burton," in Selected Writings, 88.

29. Bean, 93.

30. "Aequanimitas," in Aequanimitas, 3–7.

31. Thomas McCrae, "Osler and Patient," in Sir William Osler, Bart., 61.

32. "Alfred Stillé," in An Alabama Student, 244.

33. A. E. Rodin and J. D. Key, "William Osler and Aequanimitas: An Appraisal of His Reactions to Adversity," Journal of the Royal Society of Medicine 1994 (87): 758–763.

34. "Aequanimitas," in Aequanimitas, 11.

35. Marcia Grad, Charisma: How to Get "That Special Magic" (North Hollywood, Calif.: Wilshire, 1986), 15.

36. Ibid., 78

37. Cushing, ii, 175.

38. Joseph H. Pratt, "Aequanimitas," Arch Intern Med 1949 (84): 86–92.

39. Plutarch, "Alexander," in The Age of Alexander, translated by Ian Scott-Kilvert (London: Penguin, 1973), 299.

40. Cushing, i, 168.

41. Earl F. Nation and John P. McGovern, eds., Student and Chief: The Osler-Camac Correspondence (Pasadena, Calif.: Castle, 1980).

42. Reid, 95. See also John P. McGovern and Wilburt C. Davison, "Osler and Children," JAMA 1969 (210): 2241–2244.

43. Reid, 100.

44. Earl F. Nation, "Sir William Osler, the Master of Ewelme."

45. Cushing, ii, 188–189.

46. "Osler and the Doll Rosalie," Harvard Medical Alumni Bulletin 1949 (23): 110–113.

47. Cushing, ii, 161.

48. Palmer H. Futcher, "The Letters of William Osler to Marjorie Howard: Shared Courtship, Family, and Bereavement," Transactions and Studies of the College of Physicians of Philadelphia 1990 (12): 413–443.

49. "Dr. Johnston as a Physician," Washington Medical Annals 1902 (1): 158–161.

50. Browne, "Religio Medici," part 2, section 4, in The Prose of Sir Thomas Browne, 73–74.

51. Ibid., part 1, section 43, 51.

52. Lectures on Angina Pectoris and Allied States (New York: D. Appleton, 1897).

53. Edward H. Bensley and Donald G. Bates, "Sir William Osler's Autobiographical Notes," Bull Hist Med 1976 (50): 596–618.

54. Ibid.

55. W. Bruce Fye, "William Osler's Departure from North America: The Price of Success," in Barondess and Roland, 245–257.

56. Ibid.

57. Bensley and Bates, "Sir William Osler's Autobiographical Notes" (see note 53).

58. "On the Educational Value of the Medical Society," in Aequanimitas, 342.

59. "The Lumleian Lectures on Angina Pectoris," Lancet 1910 (1): 697–702, 839–844, 973–977.

60. "The Medical Clinic: A Retrospect and a Forecast," BMJ 1914 (1): 10–16.

61. "Chauvinism in Medicine," in Aequanimitas, 283.

62. Leon R. Kass, "The Care of the Doctor," Perspectives in Biology and Medicine 1991 (34): 553–560.

63. Betty Hosmer Mawardi, "Satisfactions, Dissatisfactions, and Causes of Stress in Medical Practice," JAMA 1979 (241): 1483–1486.

64. For brief reviews, see George Blumer, "The Jocular Side of Osler," Arch Intern Med 1949 (84): 34–38; and A. H. T. Robb-Smith, "Osler's Sense of Humour," in Oslerian Anniversary, 48–67.

65. Arthur Keith, "Osler and the Medical Museum," in Abbott, 6.

66. "Two Frenchmen on Laughter," in *Men and Books*, 9.

67. "The Student Life," in *Aequanimitas*, 405.

68. Cushing, i, 25.

69. William B. Bean, "William Osler: The Egerton Yorrick Davis Alias," in McGovern and Burns, 49–59.

70. Pratt, "Aequanimitas" (see note 38).

71. Herbert F. West, "Rabelais, Sterne and Osler: Companions in Wit," *Transactions and Studies of the College of Physicians of Philadelphia* 1959 (27): 60–73. See also Paul L. Kimmel, "François Rabelais: Satire as Therapy for the Body Politic," *Pharos* 1992 (Summer): 7–12.

72. William D. Tiggert, "An Annotated Life of Egerton Yorrick Davis, M.D., an Intimate of Sir William Osler," *Journal of the History of Medicine and Allied Sciences* 1983 (38): 259–297. See also Earl F. Nation, "Osler's Alter Ego," *Chest* 1969 (56): 531–537; and Lawrence F. Altaffer, III, "Penis Captivus and the Mischievous Sir William Osler," *Southern Medical Journal* 1983 (76): 637–641.

73. Richard L. Golden and Charles G. Roland, eds., *Sir William Osler: An Annotated Bibliography with Illustrations* (San Francisco: Norman, 1988), 179.

74. Robb-Smith, "Osler's Sense of Humour," in *Oslerian Anniversary*, 48–67.

75. Pratt, "Aequanimitas" (see note 38).

76. For another example, see Thomas S. Cullen, "The Gay of Heart," *Arch Intern Med* 1949 (84): 41–45. Osler was a classic example of what the psychologist Wayne W. Dyer calls "a person who has eliminated all erroneous zones." See Dyer, *Your Erroneous Zones* (New York: Funk & Wagnalls, 1976), 222–234.

77. Clifford Allbutt, "Sir William Osler," *Nature* 1919/1920 (104): 402.

78. Marian Osborne, "Recollections of Sir William Osler," in Abbott, 174.

79. Cullen, "The Gay of Heart" (see note 76). See also Blumer, "The Jocular Side of Osler" (note 64).

80. William Zinn, "The Empathic Physician," *Arch Intern Med* 1993 (153): 306–312. See also Howard Spiro, "What Is Empathy and Can It Be Taught?," *Ann Intern Med* 1992 (116): 843–846.

81. Full discussions of the concepts of caring and compassion far exceed the scope of this section. For an operational account of the components of caring that can be clearly identified in Osler's life, see Martin A. Adson, "An Endangered Ethic—the Capacity for Caring," *Mayo Clinic Proceedings* 1995 (70): 495–500. The terms "caring," "sympathy," and "compassion" are used somewhat loosely today. The Hippocratic notion of love for humanity that Osler was fond of quoting does not imply compassion in the sense of fellow-suffering with patients. "Compassion" may have been introduced into the medical literature as *humanitas* by a Roman writer (possibly a physician) of the first century A.D. named Scribonius Largus. *Humanitas* was distinctly different from *philanthropia*, the term used by Osler in his last major address, which conveyed "a feeling of solidarity of all men as short lived and frail subjects of fate." See Edmund D. Pellegrino, "The Virtuous Physician, and the Ethics of Medicine," in Earl E. Shelp, ed., *Virtue and Medicine: Explorations in the Character of Medicine* (Dordrecht, Holland: D. Reidel, 1985), 248; and Edmund D. Pellegrino and Alice A. Pellegrino, "Humanism and Ethics in Roman Medicine: Translation and Commentary on a Text of Scribonius Largus," in Barondess and Roland, 30–31. See also Gregory E. Pence, "Can Compassion be Taught?" *Journal of Medical Ethics* 1983 (9): 189–191.

82. See Philip W. Leon, *Walt Whitman and Sir William Osler: A Poet and His Physician* (Toronto: ECW Press, 1995); and Wilder Penfield, "Halsted of Johns Hopkins: The Man and His Problem as Described in the Secret Records of William Osler," *JAMA* 1969 (210): 2214–2218, 1989.

83. Wilder Penfield, "Neurology in Canada and the Osler Centennial," *CMAJ* 1949 (61):69–73.

84. C. E. Newman, "Osler as a Physician," in *Oslerian Anniversary*, 13–14.

85. "The Treatment of Disease," *Canada Lancet* 1909 (42): 899–912.

86. Thomas McCrae, "Osler and Patient," in *Sir William Osler, Bart.*, 61–62.

87. Cushing, i, 682.

88. W. G. MacCallum, "A Student's Impression of Osler," *CMAJ* 1920 (Sir William Osler Memorial Number, July), 47–50.

89. Aristotle, *The Nicomachean Ethics*, translated by David Ross (Oxford: Oxford University Press, 1991), 232–234.

90. Cushing, ii, 277.

91. Wilburt C. Davison, "Sir William Osler: Reminiscences," *Arch Intern Med* 1949 (84): 110–128.

92. Cushing, i, 14–15.

93. Branden calls self-esteem "the immune system of the consciousness" and suggests that there are six components: living consciously, self-acceptance, self-responsibility, self-assertiveness, living purposefully, and practicing personal integrity. See Nathaniel Branden, *The Six Pillars of Self-Esteem* (New York: Bantam, 1994). See also Matthew McKay and Patrick Fanning, *Self-Esteem*, 2d edition (Oakland, Calif.: New Harbinger, 1992).

94. Levinson defines self-esteem by the formula 1/(ego ideal minus self-image), which is to say that the wider the gap between ego ideal and self-image, the lower the self-esteem. See Levinson, *Psychological Man* (Cambridge, Mass.: Levinson Institute, 1976), 12.

95. "The Reserves of Life," *St. Mary's Hospital Gazette* 1907 (13): 95–98.

96. Detailed analysis of Osler's many-sided personality exceeds my scope and competence. However, brief considerations in currently popular frameworks may be helpful. In the framework of transactional analysis—in which personality is divided into "parent," "adult," and "child" components—Osler gave free rein to his "nourishing parent" and "happy, okay child" and knew how to maintain his "adult" while keeping his "critical parent" and "unhappy, not-okay child" at bay. See Thomas A. Harris, *I'm OK—You're OK* (New York: Avon, 1973). In the framework of the Myers-Briggs Type Inventory, Osler was able to establish good relationships with people irrespective of where they stood on the extroversion/introversion, sensing/intuiting, thinking/feeling, and judging/perceiving scales. See Isabel Briggs Myers and Peter B. Myers, *Gifts Differing* (Palo Alto, Calif.: Consulting Psychologists Press, 1980). It is telling that when his friends honored him on his seventieth birthday, the volume of tributes was subtitled "Brief Tributes to His Personality . . ." (see *Sir William Osler, Bart.*). The extent to which Osler was loved by his contemporaries is perhaps the strongest argument against the "anti-Oslerians" who arise from time to time.

97. Reinhold Niebuhr's "Serenity Prayer" (1934) reads: "God, give us grace to accept with serenity the things that cannot be changed, courage to change the things which should be changed, and the wisdom to distinguish the one from the other." Among the classic statements to this effect by the Stoic philosophers is *The Enchiridion* by Epictetus, which begins: "There are things which are within our power, and there are things which are beyond our power."

98. Cushing, i, 636–637. See also C. B. Farrar, "I Remember Osler, Psychotherapist," *American Journal of Psychiatry* 1965 (121): 761–762.

CHAPTER 7

1. Henry W. Cattell, "Osler, the Medical Editor," in Abbott, 88.

2. The most recent and definitive compilation is Richard L. Golden and Charles G. Roland, eds., *Sir William Osler: An Annotated Bibliography with Illustrations* (San Francisco: Norman, 1988).

3. For reviews of Osler as a writer, see Bett, 102–105; Edward N. Brush, "Osler's Literary Style," in *Sir William Osler, Bart.*, 115–120; William White, "The Literary Physician: A Note on Osler's Essays," *California and Western Medicine* 1941 (54): 79–80; Charles

G. Roland, "Osler's Writing Style," *JAMA* 1969 (210): 2257–2260; and Faith Wallis, "The Literary Styles of Sir William Osler," *Osler Library Newsletter* 1986 (51): 1–3.

4. *The Principles and Practice of Medicine* (New York: D. Appleton, 1892), 371.

5. Fielding H. Garrison, "Osler's Place in the History of Medicine," in Abbott, 31.

6. "The War and Typhoid Fever," *Transactions of the Society of Tropical Medicine and Hygiene* 1914 (8): 45–61.

7. "Oliver Wendell Holmes," in *An Alabama Student*, 66–67.

8. "The Pathological Institute of a General Hospital," *Glasgow Medical Journal* 1911 (5): 321–333.

9. Bean, 100, 117, 129–130, 132, 140.

10. C. F. Martin, "Osler as Clinician and Teacher," in Abbott, 44.

11. David Naylor, "Osler's First Medical Publications," *CMAJ* 1984 (131): 800–806.

12. Stewart R. Roberts, "William Osler, Clinician-Teacher," in Abbott, 434.

13. "Pathological Report," in *Montreal General Hospital: Reports Clinical and Pathological by the Medical Staff*, edited by William Osler (Montreal: Dawson Brothers, 1880), 276.

14. Bean, 56.

15. Stewart R. Roberts, "William Osler, Clinician-Teacher," in Abbott, 432.

16. Bean, 57.

17. "Dr. Johnston as a Physician," *Washington Medical Annals* 1902 (1): 158–161.

18. Bean, 76.

19. Bean, 56.

20. See Henry W. Cattell, "Osler, the Medical Editor," in Abbott, 88–90; and Charles G. Roland, "William Osler and Medical Journalism," *JAMA* 1967 (200): 386–390.

21. *The Evolution of Modern Medicine*, 154.

22. Cushing, i, 242.

23. William White, "Osler on Shakespeare, Bacon, and Burton, with a reprint of his Creators, Transmuters, and Transmitters as Illustrated by Shakespeare, Bacon, and Burton," *Bull Hist Med* 1939 (7): 392–408.

24. *Lectures on the Diagnosis of Abdominal Tumors* (New York: D. Appleton , 1898), 191.

25. William White, "Osler on Shakespeare, Bacon, and Burton" (see note 23). The quotation is from Matthew Arnold, "Shakespeare."

26. Ibid.

27. Bean, 77.

28. Bacon, *Essays*, 150.

29. Edward N. Brush, "Osler's Literary Style," in *Sir William Osler, Bart.*, 115–120.

30. Francis R. Packard, "Literary Influences on the Writings of Osler," in Abbott, 26.

31. This aphorism attributed to Osler appears on a medal designed for the Jikei Medical College, Tokyo, Japan. See Alex Sakula, *The Portraiture of Sir William Osler* (London: Royal Society of Medicine, 1991), 79–81.

32. Warfield T. Longcope, "Random Recollections of William Osler, 1899–1918," *Arch Intern Med* 1949 (84): 93–103.

33. Bean, 126.

34. William Sydney Thayer, "Reminiscences of Osler in the Early Baltimore Days," in Thayer, *Osler and Other Papers* (Freeport, N.Y.: Books for Libraries Press, 1931), 21.

35. Reid, 83–84.

36. Hiram Woods, "Influence in Building Up the Medical and Chirurgical Faculty," in *Sir William Osler, Bart.*, 90.

37. Plutarch, "On Listening," in *Essays*, 27–50.

38. Tony Alessandra, *The Dynamics of Effective Listening* (Niles, Ill.: Nightingale-Conant Corporation, 1994), audiocassette. See also Phillip L. Hunsaker and Anthony J. Alessandra, *The Art of Managing People* (New York: Simon & Schuster, 1980), 120–144.

39. Reid, 183.

40. George Blumer, "The Jocular Side of Osler," *Arch Intern Med* 1949; 84: 34–38.

41. William S. Thayer, "Osler," in Abbott, 287.

42. A. D. Blackader, "Osler's Early Work for Canadian Scientific Societies and as a Teacher in Montreal," in Abbott, 159.

43. "After Twenty-Five Years," in *Aequanimitas*, 191–193.

44. D. J. Gibb Wishart, "Osler from the Standpoint of the Undergraduate," in Abbott, 177.

45. A. Schmidt, "Student Reminiscences—Montreal Period," in Abbott, 183.

46. Cushing, i, 123.

47. J. B. Lawford, "Student Reminiscences—Montreal Period," in Abbott, 179.

48. Ralph Waldo Emerson, "Eloquence," in *Society and Solitude* (Boston: Houghton, Mifflin, 1870), 81.

49. Cushing, i, 234–235.

50. Charles W. Burr, "Some Personal Reminiscences of Sir William Osler in Philadelphia," in Abbott, 222–223.

51. Joseph Leidy, 2d, "Student Reminiscences—Philadelphia Period," in Abbott, 218.

52. George Dock, "Dr. William Osler in Philadelphia, 1884–1889," in Abbott, 210.

53. J. M. T. Finney, "A Personal Appreciation of Sir William Osler," in Abbott, 278.

54. William S. Thayer, "Osler," in Abbott, 287.

55. Stewart R. Roberts, "William Osler, Clinician-Teacher," in Abbott, 433.

56. Cushing, ii, 338–339.

57. Ibid., i, 182.

58. "Vienna After Thirty-Four Years," *JAMA* 1908 (50): 1523–1525.

59. Cushing, ii, 648–649.

60. Ibid., 351–352.

61. Browne, "Religio Medici," part 2, section 10, in *The Prose of Sir Thomas Browne*, 82.

62. "Dr. Johnston as a Physician" (see note 17).

63. Edgar Lorrington Gilcreest, "Sir William Osler—Physician and Philanthropist—Glimpses During the World War," in Abbott, 414.

64. Cushing, i, 354–355.

65. Cushing, ii, 356.

66. "The Student Life," in *Aequanimitas*, 417.

67. "The Leaven of Science," in *Aequanimitas*, 79–81.

68. Cushing, ii, 407.

69. "The Army Surgeon," in *Aequanimitas*, 102.

70. D. Bryson Delavan, "A Reminiscence of Sir William Osler," in Abbott, 204.

71. H. A. Lafleur, "Early Days at The Johns Hopkins Hospital with Dr. Osler," in Abbott, 272.

72. Reid, 133.

73. William S. Thayer, "Osler," in Abbott, 292.

74. See Ralph Waldo Emerson, "Clubs," in *Society and Solitude* (Boston and New York: Houghton, Mifflin, 1870), 223–250.

75. A. G. Gibson, "Sir William Osler at Oxford: A Personal Reminiscence," in Abbott, 379.

76. Sakula, "Sir William Osler and the Royal Society of Medicine, London," in Barondess and Roland, 179–182.

77. Cushing, ii, 34–35.

78. Ibid., 129–130, 141.

79. Norman B. Gwyn, "The Medical Arena in the Toronto of Osler's Early Days in the Study of Medicine," *Arch Intern Med* 1949 (84): 2–6.

80. Edward N. Brush, "Osler's Influence on Other Medical Schools in Baltimore: His Relation to the Medical Profession," in *Sir William Osler, Bart.*, 85.

81. Humphry Rolleston, "Sir William Osler in Great Britain," in Abbott, 349.

82. A. Schmidt, "Student Reminiscences—Montreal Period," in Abbott, 183.

83. "Rudolph Virchow, the Man and the Student," *Boston Medical and Surgical Journal* 1891 (125): 425–427.

84. "The Student Life," in *Aequanimitas*, 416–417.

85. "The Future of the Medical Profession in Canada. Address before the Medical Society of the C.A.M.C., Shorncliffe, Sept. 9th, 1918." Unpublished manuscript. Osler Library of the History of Medicine, McGill University, Montreal.

86. Oliver Wendell Holmes, "The Young Practitioner," in *Medical Essays, 1842–1882* (Boston: Houghton, Mifflin, 1883), 384.

87. Philip K. Bondy, "What's So Special About Osler?" *Yale Journal of Biology and Medicine* 1980 (53): 213–217.

88. William S. Thayer, "Osler," in Abbott, 291.

89. Pratt, vi-vii.

90. For this and other examples, see Charles R. Roland, "Osler's Rough Edge," in Barondess, McGovern, and Roland, 39–43.

91. Ibid.

92. Cushing, i, 423–424. See also Richard L. Golden, ed., *Oslerian Verse: An Annotated Anthology* (Montreal: Osler Library, McGill University, 1992), 24–27.

93. George M. Kober, "The Influence of Dr. Osler on American Medicine," in Abbott, 55.

94. [William H. Welch], "William Osler," in *Papers and Addresses by William Henry Welch* (Baltimore: Johns Hopkins Press, 1920), 451–452.

95. J. M. T. Finney, "A Personal Appreciation of Sir William Osler," in Abbott, 275.

96. Joseph H. Pratt, "Osler as His Students Knew Him," *Boston Medical and Surgical Journal* 1920 (182): 338–341.

97. Francis J. Shepherd, "Osler's Montreal Period: A Personal Reminiscence," in Abbott, 156.

98. Stewart P. Roberts, "William Osler, Clinician-Teacher," in Abbott, 432.

99. Cushing, ii, 92.

100. "Nurse and Patient," in *Aequanimitas*, 153.

101. William S. Thayer, "Osler, the Teacher," in *Sir William Osler, Bart.*, 52.

102. "Internal Medicine as a Vocation," in *Aequanimitas*, 144.

103. W. W. Francis, "Osler and the Reporters, with an Unpublished Note on 'The Fixed Period,' " *CMAJ* 1949 (61): 68–69.

104. "The Fixed Period," in *Aequanimitas*, 376–377. See also William B. Bean, "Osler, Trollope and the Fixed Period," *Transactions of the American Clinical and Climatological Association* 1966 (78): 242–248; and Horton A. Johnson, "Osler Recommends Chloroform at Sixty," *Pharos* 1996 (Winter): 24–26..

105. Ibid., 381–383.

106. Francis, "Osler and the Reporters" (see note 103).

107. Cushing, i, 668–669.

108. Preface, in *Aequanimitas*, viii.

109. Steven L. Berk, "Sir William Osler, Ageism, and 'The Fixed Period': A Secret Revealed," in Barondess and Roland, 297–301.

110. Joseph H. Pratt, "Aequanimitas," *Arch Intern Med* 1949 (84): 86–92.

111. Wilburt C. Davison, "Sir William Osler: Reminiscences," *Arch Intern Med* 1949 (84): 110–128.

CHAPTER 8

1. "L'Envoi," in *Aequanimitas*, 451.

2. Bean, 94.

3. W. S. Thayer, "Osler, The Teacher," in *Sir William Osler, Bart.*, 53.

4. "The Evolution of the Idea of Experiment in Medicine," in *Transactions of the*

Congress of American Physicians and Surgeons, Seventh Triennial Session (New Haven, Conn.: By the Congress, 1907), 7.

5. "The Reserves of Life," *St. Mary's Hospital Gazette* 1907 (13): 95–98.

6. "A Way of Life," in *Selected Writings*, 245.

7. Bean, 95.

8. Ibid.

9. Ibid., 94–95.

10. Ibid., 66.

11. "A Way of Life," in *Selected Writings*, 245.

12. Ibid.

13. Bean, 96.

14. Cushing, ii, 23.

15. "Unity, Peace, and Concord," in *Aequanimitas*, 437.

16. Lewellys F. Barker, "Dr. Osler as the Young Physician's Friend and Exemplar," in Abbott, 255.

17. Henry Barton Jacobs, "Osler in Vacation," in Abbott, 92–93.

18. Cushing, i, 111.

19. C. F. Martin, "Osler as Clinician and Teacher," in *Sir William Osler Memorial Number, CMAJ,* July 1920, 82–87.

20. Edward H. Bentley and Donald G. Bates, "Sir William Osler's Autobiographical Notes," *Bull Hist Med* 1976 (50): 596–618.

21. Charles G. Roland, "Sir William Osler's Dreams and Nightmares," *Bull Hist Med* 1980 (54): 418–446.

22. Richard L. Golden, "Sir William Osler's Angina Pectoris and Other Disorders," *American Journal of Cardiology* 1987 (60): 175–178.

23. Bacon, *Essays*, 98–99.

24. Cushing, ii, 83.

25. "Dr. Osler's Recipe for a Life of Happiness," *Abingdon* [England] *Herald*, November 24, 1906. See also *The Times* [London], November 20, 1906.

26. Bean, 49.

27. Rudyard Kipling usually receives credit for "He travels fastest who travels alone."

28. "The Master-Word in Medicine," in *Aequanimitas*, 364–365.

29. "Nurse and Patient," in *Aequanimitas*, 155.

30. Browne, "Religio Medici," part 2, section 9, in *The Prose of Sir Thomas Browne*, 80.

31. "A Way of Life," in *Selected Writings*, 245.

32. Cervantes, part 1, book 3, chapter 10, 211.

33. "Internal Medicine as a Vocation," in *Aequanimitas*, 136. See also G. Stout, "Who Was Dr Lydgate?" *Journal of Medical Biography* 1996 (4):100–101.

34. Bean, 66.

35. George T. Harrell, "Osler's Professorships and His Families," *Perspectives in Biology and Medicine* 1985 (29 [1]): 76–87.

36. Thomas E. Keys, "Osler's Librarian, Dr. W. W. Francis," in Barondess, McGovern, and Roland, 213–222.

37. Cushing, i, 264.

38. Ibid., 357–358.

39. Francis R. Packard, "William Osler in Philadelphia, 1884–1889," *Arch Intern Med* 1949 (84): 18–25.

40. J.M.T. Finney, "A Personal Appreciation of Sir William Osler," in Abbott, 282.

41. Archibald Malloch, "Sir William Osler at Oxford," in Abbott, 375.

42. Frederick B. Wagner, Jr., *The Twilight Years of Lady Osler: Letters of a Doctor's Wife* (Canton, Mass.: Science History Publications, 1985).

43. Cushing, ii, 137.

44. Joseph H. Pratt, "Osler as his Students Knew Him," *Boston Medical and Surgical Journal* 1920 (14): 338–341.

45. Cushing, ii, 642.

46. George T. Harrell, "Lady Osler," in Barondess, McGovern, and Roland, 19–34.

47. George T. Harrell, "The Oslers' Son—Revere," in Barondess and Roland, 259–268.

48. Cushing, ii, 577–578.

49. Ibid., i, 175.

50. Howard L. Holley, *A Continual Remembrance: Letters from Sir William Osler to his friend Ned Milburn, 1865–1919* (Springfield, Ill.: Charles C Thomas, 1968).

51. Cushing, i, 24–25.

52. Ibid., 157–158.

53. Lewellys F. Barker, "Dr. Osler as the Young Physician's Friend and Exemplar," in Abbott, 257.

54. William Hale-White, "Appreciation of Sir William Osler," in Abbott, 356.

55. Cushing, ii, 209.

56. "After Twenty-Five Years," in *Aequanimitas*, 195–196.

57. "Samuel Wilks," in *Men and Books*, 6.

58. Reid, 66.

59. Daniel J. Levinson, *The Seasons of a Man's Life* (New York: Alfred A. Knopf, 1978), 335. See also David W. Smith, *The Friendless American Male* (Ventura, Calif.: Regal Books, 1983).

60. Aristotle, *Nichomachean Ethics*, translated by David Ross (Oxford: Oxford University Press, 1991), books 8 and 9, 192–247.

61. Plutarch, "How to Distinguish a Flatterer from a Friend," in *Essays*, 61–112.

62. Montaigne, "Of Friendship," in *The Complete Works of Montaigne*, 135–144.

63. Emerson, "Friendship," in *Essays*, 159–180.

64. For a contemporary review of the literature on friendship, see Neera Kapur Badhwar, ed., *Friendship: A Philosophical Reader* (Ithaca: Cornell University Press, 1993).

65. F. H. Garrison, "Sir William Osler (1849–1919)," *Science* 1920; 51 (new series): 55–58.

66. "Chauvinism in Medicine," in *Aequanimitas*, 285.

67. "The Master-Word in Medicine," in *Aequanimitas*, 365.

68. "After Twenty-Five Years," in *Aequanimitas*, 203–204.

69. J. M. T. Finney, "A Personal Appreciation of Sir William Osler," in Abbott, 279–280.

70. "The Medical Library in Post-Graduate Work," *BMJ* 1909 (2): 925–928.

71. Cushing, ii, 586.

72. "After Twenty-Five Years," in *Aequanimitas*, 205.

73. "British Medicine in Greater Britain," in *Aequanimitas*, 168–169.

74. "The Master-Word in Medicine," in *Aequanimitas*, 366–367.

75. "The Student Life," in *Aequanimitas*, 414.

76. "The Collecting of a Library," in *Selected Writings*, 263–266.

77. A. C. Abbott, "Student Reminiscences—Johns Hopkins Period," in Abbott, 304. See also Leonard Payne, "Osler as a Bibliophile," in *Oslerian Anniversary*, 38–47.

78. Henry Barton Jacobs, "Osler in Vacation," in Abbott, 9.

79. Ibid., 92–94.

80. William Hale-White, "Appreciation of Sir William Osler," in Abbott, 352.

81. Cushing, ii, 102–103.

82. Ibid., 132.

83. "The Leaven of Science," in *Aequanimitas*, 90.

84. *Man's Redemption of Man* (New York: Paul B. Hoeber, 1913), 28–29.

85. Browne, "Religio Medici," part 1, section 27, in *The Prose of Sir Thomas Browne*, 35.

86. Ibid., section 1, 7.

87. "Sir Thomas Browne," in *An Alabama Student*, 273.

88. *The Evolution of Modern Medicine*, 2.

89. Cushing, ii, 298.

90. Browne, "Religio Medici," part 2, section 11, in *The Prose of Sir Thomas Browne*, 85.

91. Ibid., part 1, section 45, 52.

92. Ibid., section 52, 60.

93. *Science and Immortality* (Boston: Houghton, Mifflin, 1904). For brief commentary and excerpts from the lecture, see Nathaniel Edward Griffin and Lawrence Hunt, eds., *The Farther Shore: An Anthology of World Opinion on the Immortality of the Soul* (Boston: Houghton Mifflin, 1934), 265–274.

94. William White, "*Æquanimitas*: Osler's Inspirational Essays," *Bull Hist Med* 1938 (6): 820–833.

95. Ludwig Edelstein, "William Osler's Philosophy," *Bull Hist Med* 1946 (20): 270–293.

96. "The Treatment of Disease," *Canada Lancet* 1909 (42): 899–912.

97. "The Master-Word in Medicine," in *Aequanimitas*, 365.

98. Archibald Malloch, "Sir William Osler at Oxford," in Abbott, 365.

99. Cushing, ii, 224.

100. Palmer Howard Futcher, "William Osler's Religion," *Arch Intern Med* 1961 (107): 475-479.

101. "Robert Burton," in *Selected Writings*, 87.

102. *The Evolution of Modern Medicine*, 62.

103. "Medicine in the Nineteenth Century," in *Aequanimitas*, 258–260.

104. "The Faith That Heals," *BMJ* 1910 (2): 1470–1472.

105. Edmund J. A. Rogers, "Personal Reminiscences of the Earlier Years of Sir William Osler," in Abbott, 164.

106. Julius Seelye Bixler, "The Existentialists and William James," *American Scholar* 1958–1959 (28 [1]): 83.

107. "The Old Humanities and the New Science," in *Selected Writings*, 29.

108. Thomas McCrae, "The Influence of Pathology on the Clinical Medicine of William Osler," in Abbott, 40.

109. "Teacher and Student," in *Aequanimitas*, 40–41.

110. "L'Envoi," in *Aequanimitas*, 451.

111. Cushing, i, 8–9.

112. The four sons whose careers were exceptional were Featherston, who served as justice of the Court of Appeal for Ontario for 31 years and then as a corporation president; Britton Bath ("B. B."), known throughout Canada as "the thirteenth juryman" by virtue of his reputation as a leading trial attorney; Edmund Boyd ("E. B."), who headed one of Canada's leading brokerage firms, served as a bank president and as a director of many companies, and was knighted; and William. The other brothers were Edward Lake, an attorney; and Francis Lewellyn ("Frank"), whose difficulties in life were attributed by his mother to her inadequate supply of milk. For a warmly written history of the family, see Anne Wilkinson, *Lions in the Way: A Discursive History of the Oslers* (Toronto: Macmillan, 1956).

113. Cushing, i, 294.

114. "The Master-Word in Medicine," in *Aequanimitas*, 368–369.

115. "Teaching and Thinking," in *Aequanimitas*, 118.

116. Cushing, ii, 443.

117. Wilburt C. Davison, "Sir William Osler: Reminiscences," *Arch Intern Med* 1949 (84): 110–128. See also Alfred R. Henderson, "War Comes to the Peacemaker: William Osler, 1914–1918," *Military Medicine* 1971 (136): 227–233.

118. George William Norris, "Sir William Osler as Host to Americans in England During the War," in Abbott, 408.

119. Hobart Amory Hare, "William Osler as a Teacher and Clinician in Philadelphia," in Abbott, 217.

120. J. M. T. Finney, "A Personal Appreciation of Sir William Osler," in Abbott, 284–285.

121. J. George Adami, "Sir William Osler: The Last Days," in Abbott, 422–423.

122. Shigeaki Hinohara, "Sir William Osler's Philosophy on Death," *Ann Intern Med* 1993 (118): 638–642.

123. Cushing, ii, 679.

EPILOGUE

1. See E. Rosencrantz, "Posthumous Tributes to Sir William Osler," *Arch Intern Med* 1949 (84): 170–197; Earl F. Nation, Charles G. Roland, and John P. McGovern, *An Annotated Checklist of Osleriana* (Kent, Ohio: Kent State University Press, 1976); Richard L. Golden, "Medallic Tributes to Sir William Osler and Their Historical Associations," *JAMA* 1979 (242): 2862–2867; Alex Sakula, *The Portraiture of Sir William Osler* (London: Royal Society of Medicine, 1991); and Richard L. Golden, ed., *Oslerian Verse: An Annotated Anthology* (Montreal: Osler Library, McGill University, 1992).

2. Alvin E. Rodin and Jack D. Key, "Osler's Brain and Related Mental Matters," in Barondess and McGovern, 303–312.

3. Browne, "A Letter to a Friend," in *The Prose of Sir Thomas Browne*, 362.

4. "A Way of Life," in *Selected Writings*, 239.

Index

Addison, Thomas, 63
Aequanimitas, 134, 141, 143, 158. *See also* Equanimity
Allbutt, Thomas Clifford, 155, 191–92
Ambition, personal, 8, 10, 22
Antoninus Pius, 143
Aristotle, 20, 68, 129, 158, 213
Association of American Physicians, 180
Association of Physicians of Great Britain and Ireland, 49
Atkinson, William Biddle, 180
Attitude, value of positive, 83–87

Bacon, Francis, 44, 165–66, 192
Baltimore, Maryland, 16, 55, 178–79, 180–81. *See also* Osler, William, at The Johns Hopkins University (Baltimore period)
Barker, Lewellys Franklin, 50, 199
Bartlett, Elisha, 10, 71, 120, 204
Bassett, John Y., 56–57
Bean, William Bennett, 113
Beaumont, William, 39–40
Belfast, Northern Ireland, 125
Berlin, Germany, 10, 41, 119

Bern, Switzerland, 36
Bernard, Claude, 130
Bett, Walter Reginald, 41
Billings, John Shaw, 96
Bly, Robert, 60
Boerhaave, Hermann, 127
Bovell, James, 33–34, 60–61, 63–66, 69, 71, 72, 73, 79–80
Branden, Nathaniel, 159
Bright, Richard, 63
Brödel, Max, 155
Browne, Thomas, 7, 88, 94, 115, 157, 167, 176, 183, 199, 203, 213
   on charity to oneself, 147
   on goals, 9
   on habits, 18
   on interpersonal relations, 97–98, 101–2, 119, 174–75
   as "lifelong mentor" to William Osler, 5, 31, 62, 67–68, 186, 218
   as optimist, 84
   on passion, 193–94
   as philosopher of religion, 34, 206–7, 208
   as skeptic, 119–20
   on virtue, 39, 218–19

Brush, Edward N., 166
Bunyan, John, 14
Burton, Robert, 83, 140, 199
Butler, Bishop Joseph, 122

Caldwell, Charles, 176
Camac, Charles Nicoll Bancker, 75–76, 145
Campbell, Joseph, 31–32
Canadian Medical Association, 48, 115, 137, 173–74
Caring, methods and nature of, 133–60, 244–45 n. 81
  for oneself, 147–51
Carlyle, Thomas, 5, 14, 183
Carroll, Lewis [Charles Ludwidge Dodgson], 158
Cervantes Saavedra, Miguel de, 101–2, 168, 194
Character, definitions of, 20, 218 fig., 219
Charisma, components of, 144–47
Churchill, Winston Leonard Spenser, 178
Communication, skills of, 161–86
Compassion. See Caring
Cosmopolitanism, value of, 36–37, 41–43
Courage, as value, 212–16
Covey, Stephen R., 23, 53
Cowper, William, 116
Cushing, Harvey
  as biographer of William Osler, 15, 21, 26, 27, 54, 61, 62, 65, 67, 73, 77, 81, 144, 157, 172, 175, 182
  as protégé of William Osler, 80

Darwin, Charles Robert, 33, 206
Day-tight compartments, 4, 6, 13–17
Decisiveness, as trait, 23, 94–96
Defense mechanisms, psychological, 100–104, 151
Descartes, René, 159
Dock, George, 25–26, 173
Drummond, William Henry, 151
Dubos, René Jules, 85
Dundas, Ontario, 5, 217
Dyer, Wayne W., 244 n. 76

Edinburgh, University of, 178
Education, process and standards of, 7, 36–37, 75, 105–31
Egypt, ancient, medicine in, 45
Einstein, Albert, 206
Eliot, Charles William, 208

Eliot, George [Mary Ann Evans], 194
Emerson, Ralph Waldo, 48, 84, 86, 172
  on friendship, 200–202
  on principles, 8
Epicharmus, 121
Epictetus, 87, 101, 168, 246 n. 97
Equanimity, value of, 8, 140–43
Erasmus, Desiderius, 69, 112
Erikson, Erik Homburger, 32

Faith, value of, 139, 211–12
Family, importance of, 193–98
Ferriar, John, 126
Finney, John Miller Turpin, 29, 173, 182, 196, 215
Francis, Marian Osler, 195
Francis, William Willoughby, 195
Franklin, Benjamin, 95
Friendships, importance of, 198–202

Galen, 69, 139
Gallio, Junius, 208–9
Garrison, Fielding Hudson, 3, 99, 202
Garth, Samuel, 53
Gates, Frederick Taylor, 17, 117
Generosity, as trait, 88–90
Gibson, Alexander George, 191–92
Gilman, Daniel Coit, 105–6
Gladstone, William Ewart, 145
Glasgow, Scotland, 163
Goal setting, value of, 8–12 (fig. 1.1, 9)
Grad, Marcia, 144
Graves, Robert James, 63
Greece, ancient. See also Hippocrates; Hippocratic ideal
  medicine, 45–46, 69, 110
  philosophy, 68, 128, 129
Green, John Richard, 121
Gross, Grace Revere. See Osler, Grace Linzee Revere
Gross, Samuel David, 115, 195
Gross, Samuel Weissell, 94, 195

Habits, value of, 4, 14–15. See also Method
Halsted, William Stewart, 156
Harvard University, 40, 207–10
Harvey, William, 69–70, 75, 125, 203
Health, importance of, 147–51, 188–93
Hebrew tradition, medicine in, 45
Herbert, George, 92
Hero-myth, universal, 31–32 (32 fig. 2.1)

Heroes, value of, 10, 67–72
Hippocrates, 68, 70
  as father of medicine, 46, 110, 111, 122
Hippocratic ideal, 133, 160
History, appreciation of, 44–48
Hobbies, importance of, 202–5
Hobbs, Charles R., 18–19
Holmes, Oliver Wendell, 72, 120
  as bedside teacher, 127
  on dangers of outside interests, 180
  as literary physician, 71, 163
  as therapeutic nihilist, 122
Honesty, intellectual, 118–23
Howard, Robert Palmer, 10, 60–61, 64–
    66, 69, 72, 73, 79–80, 135
Humor, importance of, 151–56
Hunter, John, 46, 75, 113, 129–30
Hurd, Henry Mills, 17, 48–49
Huxley, Thomas Henry, 33

Idealism, 37–41, 57, 213
Imhotep, 45
Inter-Urban Clinical Club, 131

Jacobs, Henry Barton, 205
James, William, 23, 210–11, 212
Jefferson Medical College, 196
Jenner, Edward, 129–30
Johns Hopkins Hospital, 25, 75, 105–6
Johns Hopkins University, 105–6, 184.
    See also Osler, William, at The
    Johns Hopkins University (Balti-
    more period)
  School of Medicine, 75, 96, 123–24,
    127
Johnson, William Arthur, 5, 34, 60–63,
    65, 66, 69, 72, 73
  Criticisms of William Osler, 79, 234 *n*. 70
Jung, Carl Gustav, 32

Keats, John, 25, 181
Kelly, Howard Atwood, 89, 97
Kipling, Rudyard, 39
Koch, Robert, 93, 120–21

Laennec, René, 130
Lafleur, Henri Amadée, 25
Laveran, Alphonse, 121
Legacy, value of, 53–57
Leipzig, Germany, 95
Levinson, Daniel Jacob, 32, 78, 200
Levinson, Harry, 159

Libraries, importance of, 54–56, 108–9
Life, balanced, ideal of, 67, 187–216 (fig.
    8.1, 188)
Life cycle, adult, 32–33
Linacre, Thomas, 68–70
Lincoln, Abraham, 84, 113
Listening, as skill, 167–70
Lister, Joseph, 75, 120
Locke, Charles F. A., 198
Locke, John, 34, 71, 99–100, 111, 122
London, England, 10, 29, 37, 41
  Medical Society of, 178
Louis, Pierre Charles Alexandre, 111, 130

MacCallum, William George, 111–12,
    120, 152–53
MacDonnell, Richard Lea, 25–26, 93
Marcus Aurelius, Antoninus, 87, 101, 168
Maryland State Medical Society, 76
McCrae, Thomas, 143
McGill University, 25, 60, 79, 80, 127.
    See also Osler, William, at McGill
    University (Montreal period)
Medical societies. *See* Organizations
Medicine, as profession, 35–37, 42–44.
    See also under Osler, William; and
    Osler, William, opinion
Medicine, as science. *See* Osler, William,
    opinions, on medicine as science
Menninger, Karl Augustus, 87
Mentoring, 59–81, 123–127
Method, value of, 17–21. *See also* Habits
Michaelangelo Buonarroti, 204
Milburn, Edward Fairfax (Ned), 152, 198
Milton, John, 107, 167
Minnesota, University of, 35, 118
Mitchell, Silas Weir, 95–96
Montaigne, Michel Eyquem de, 200–202
Montreal, Canada, 16, 54, 55, 152. *See*
    also Osler, William, at McGill Uni-
    versity (Montreal period)
Montreal General Hospital, 164
Musser, John Herr, 150

New Haven Medical Association, 39, 52,
    149
New York Academy of Medicine, 127
New York City, 6, 76
Niebuhr, Reinhold, 159, 246 *n*. 97
Nightingale, Earl, 84
Noble, Iris, 28, 65

Observation, in medicine, 109–15
Optimism, as personality trait, 84–87
Organizations, value of, 48–53
Osborne, Marian Georgina Francis (May), 18, 26, 88
Osler Library of the History of Medicine, McGill University, 54–56
Osler, Britton Bath (B. B.), 4, 191, 255 n. 112
Osler, Charlotte Elizabeth (Chattie), 5
Osler, Edmund Boyd (E. B.), 10, 255 n. 112
Osler, Edward Lake, 255 n. 112
Osler, Edward Revere, 197–98
    birth, 197
    childhood, 60, 197
    death, 103, 187, 197–98, 215–16
    hobbies, 197, 205
    relationship to his father, 197–98
    service in World War I, 40, 103, 197–98
Osler, Ellen Free Pickton, 85, 159, 214, 255 n. 112
Osler, Emma Henrietta, 85
Osler, Featherston, 5, 255 n. 112
Osler, Featherstone Lake, 60, 85, 152, 159, 213–14
Osler, Francis Lewellyn (Frank), 255 n. 112
Osler, Grace Linzee Revere, 96, 149, 180, 195–97
    family background, 195
    as hostess, 177
    marriage to Samuel W. Gross, 195
    marriage to William Osler, 73, 177, 195–97
Osler, Jennette, 140, 195
Osler, Marian. See Francis, Marian Osler
Osler, Paul Revere, 197
Osler, William
    alter ego, Egerton Yorrick Davis, 153–55, 163
    ambitions, 8–12, 22, 33, 204
    ancestry, 41
    aphorisms, 163–64
    as bedside teacher, 127–28
    as bibliophile, 54–56, 63–64, 73, 108–9, 199, 203–4
    birth and naming, 159
    career decisions, 9–11, 33–35, 94–96, 149
    childhood and youth, 5–6, 60–63, 163, 192
    as clinician, 156, 159–60, 212–13
    as diagnostician, 111–12
    consultation (office) practice, 11, 26–27, 117, 134–35, 147–50, 182, 196
    experiences burnout, 147–50
    hospital practice, 18, 27, 91, 117, 136, 139–40, 211
    as college student, 33, 63–64
    as communicator, 161–86
    death, 187, 215–16
    as educator, 88, 105–31, 170
    families, 41, 193, 195–98, 255 n. 112
    as father, 60, 197–98, 205
    in "fixed period" controversy, 183–86
    as friend of children, 18, 144, 146–47, 176
    as friend of elderly persons, 59, 67, 135–36, 176
    friendships, 24, 59, 76–78, 198–200
    German influence on, 41, 130, 228 n. 35
    gives Ingersoll Lecture at Harvard University, 207–10
    gives Silliman Lectures at Yale University, 47
    as hero worshiper, 67. See also Osler, William, mentors
    as historian, 44–48, 137
    as humanist, 99, 133, 137–40, 159–60, 211, 219
    as husband, 195–97
    as idealist, 4–8, 37–41, 106, 213
    illnesses of, 147–48, 187, 191–92, 215–16
    at The Johns Hopkins University (Baltimore period), 36, 54, 72, 96, 123–24, 127, 184–86
        accepts chair of medicine, 96
        reminiscences, 105–6
        reminiscences by other persons, 18, 26, 27, 49, 54, 90
        writes textbook of medicine, 16–17, 25–26, 195–96
    legacies, 17, 54–57
    and libraries, 54–56
    marriage, 73, 177, 195–97
    as Master of Ewelme, 135–136, 146
    at McGill University (Montreal period), 10–11, 54, 72, 90–91, 95–96, 127, 182
        Osler Library of the History of Medicine, as legacy, 54–56
    as pathologist, 10, 91, 164–65

reminiscences, 76, 118, 171
reminiscences by other persons, 88–
    89, 171–72, 179, 199
as teacher, 19, 88, 91, 171–72
as medical student, 5, 10, 34, 63–66
as mentor, 72–76, 80–81, 145
mentors, 5, 34, 60–72. *See also*
    Browne, Thomas
as organization member, 24, 48–53
at Oxford University (Oxford period),
    54–56, 75–76, 174, 177, 211, 218
    accepts regius professorship, 96, 149
    as Master of Ewelme, 135–36
    reminiscences by other persons, 17–
        18, 21, 90, 176
as pathologist, 65–66, 91, 111–12,
    212–13
philosophy, 87
    pragmatism, 4
    stoicism, 84, 102, 159
    views on religion, 205–12
as physician. *See* Osler, William, as
    clinician; as pathologist; as psycho-
    therapist
as politician, 178–82
as postgraduate student in Europe and
    British Isles, 10, 41, 61, 66
pranks, 5, 34, 152–56, 196–97, 198
principles and ideals, 4–8, 73–74, 106,
    219
as psychotherapist, 139, 159–60, 242
    n. 21
as role model, 3, 134
as speaker, 37–38, 171–74
as therapeutic nihilist, 120, 122–23
at University of Pennsylvannia (Philadel-
    phia period), 54, 72, 77, 140–43
    accepts chair of clinical medicine, 10–
        11, 95–96, 103, 172
    reminiscences, 76–77, 95–96
    reminiscences by other persons, 29,
        54, 103, 172–73
vacations, 204–5
in World War I, 162–63, 215
as writer, 16–17, 25–26, 161–67
Osler, William, characteristics and traits
    appearance, 18, 83, 86, 94, 144, 172
    charisma, 103, 144–47
    as conversationalist, 27, 144–45,
        167–68
    as correspondent, 27, 145
    courage, 91, 214–16

friendliness, 144–45, 174–78, 197,
    198–200
    ability to balance work and social
        activities, 15–16, 21, 23–24, 27,
        92–93
    ability to relate to a wide variety of
        people, 140, 175–76, 202
    as club member, 135, 177
    generosity, 54, 77, 88–90, 124, 199
    industry, 15–21, 26–27, 90–94, 167,
        202
    as listener, 167–68
    optimism, 83–87, 103–4
    personality, analysis, 246 *n.* 96
    rough edges, 119, 143, 157, 180–81,
        250 *n.* 90
    sense of humor, 4–5, 15, 78, 151–56,
        198
    tolerance, 49–50, 97–100
Osler, William, opinions. *See also specific*
    topics
    on aging, effect on creativity, 74, 125,
        184–86
    on brevity, 27, 173
    on caring, 133–60
    on character, definition of, 20, 219
    on competition and quarrels among phy-
        sicians, 39, 52, 87, 99, 230 *n.* 81
    on cosmopolitanism, 36–37, 41–43,
        47–48
    on courage, 6, 213
    on day-tight compartments, 13–17, 26–
        30, 34, 219
    on detachment, 18, 22–23, 93
    on education, 7, 36–37, 54, 75, 105–31
        as lifelong process, 37, 106
    on equanimity, 85, 102, 138, 140–43
    on faith, value of, 139, 211–12
    on full-time clinical faculty, 117–18
    on generalism versus specialism, 43–44
    on habits (method), 4, 14–15, 18–21,
        219
    on happiness, 65, 84, 87, 106
    on healthy lifestyle, 188–93
    on history, value of, 44–48
    on hobbies, 55, 202–5
    on human nature, 22, 40–41, 103,
        151–52
    on humanities in medicine, 69, 107
    on humility, 18, 118–19, 206–7
    on hurry sickness, 18
    on idealism, 6–7, 37–41, 57, 213

Osler, William, opinions (*continued*)
  on intellectual honesty, 118–23
  on libraries, 54–56, 108–9
  on marriage, 193–95
  on medicine, practice of, 70, 106, 109–
    18, 156–57, 167
    attention to details in, 19, 35, 110–15
    commercialism in, 11–12, 53, 137,
      241 *n*. 4
    ideals necessary for, 12, 38
    purpose of, 35–37, 38
    trials and tribulations of, 12, 28, 37,
      149–51
  on medicine, professionalism in, 39–43,
    47–48, 51–53, 71–73, 87, 99
    as career choice and calling, 35–37,
      38–41, 137
    as charitable enterprise, 137–40,
      156–57
    as exemplified by historical figures,
      67–72
    standards for physicians, 54
    as worldwide profession, 42–43, 47–
      48, 51
  on medicine, as science, 129–31
    historical perspectives on, 69–72, 93,
      129–30
    methods of, 35, 109–15, 129–31
    promise for humanity, 42, 52, 163
  on nationalism, dangers of, 42, 47
  on news media, 121, 183–86
  on observation, 109–15
  on organizations, 48–53
  on patients' rights, 138
  on priorities, 11–12, 21–26, 29, 200,
    202–3
  on punctuality, 20, 64, 93, 173
  on reading, 8, 20, 125–26, 204
  on religious attitudes and beliefs, 67,
    205–12
  on science, pros and cons of, 40–41
  on self-examination, 159
  on stress as cause of illness, 101,
    147–51
  on students, 73–74
  on student–teacher relationship, 75–76,
    123–27. *See also* Osler, William, as
    mentor
  on success, 34, 65
  on taciturnity, 84, 173, 182–86
  on temperance, 189–92
  on tenacity of will, 11

  on time management, 4–30
  on tolerance, 84–85
  on travel. *See* Osler, William, opinions,
    on cosmopolitanism
  on universities, 106–9
  on wisdom, 116–17
  on women in medicine, 36, 75, 233 *n*. 55
  on work, 4, 7, 34, 84, 90–94
Osler, William, selected writings,
  "Aequanimitas," 134, 138, 140–43
  Aequanimitas collection of essays, 72,
    105, 185–86
  "A Backwood Physiologist," 39–40
  Bibliotheca Osleriana, 56
  The Evolution of Modern Medicine, 47
  "The Fixed Period," 184–86
  *The Old Humanities and the New Sci-
    ence*, 174
  The Principles and Practice of Medicine,
    60, 78–79, 115, 162, 218
    impact of, 16–17
    writing of, 16–17, 25–26, 31, 195–96
  Science and Immortality, 207–10
  "The War and Typhoid Fever," 162–63
  "A Way of Life," 29–30
Oxford, England, 6. *See also* Osler, Wil-
  liam, at Oxford University (Oxford
  period)
Oxford University, 55, 88. *See also* Osler,
  William, at Oxford University (Ox-
  ford period)

Packard, Francis Randolph, 166–67
Paget, Sir James, 35
Paley, William, 61, 80
Pareto principle, 23
Paris, France, 10, 41, 196–97
Parvin, Theophilus, 153
Pasteur, Louis, 40, 75
Peale, Norman Vincent, 84
Penfield, Wilder Graves, 21
Pennsylvania, University of, 75. *See also*
  Osler, William, at University of
  Pennsylvania (Philadelphia period)
Pepper, Oliver Hazard Perry, 74
Pepper, William, 10, 71, 72, 74, 103, 150
Philadelphia, Pennsylvania, 16, 55. *See
  also* Osler, William, at University of
  Pennsylvania (Philadelphia period)
Plato, 22, 46, 129, 199, 210
  on education, 6, 203
  on medicine, 123

Plutarch, 145, 199
  on character, 20, 219
  on friendship, 200–201
  on listening, 168–70
Politics, value of, 178–82
Pratt, Joseph Hersey, 134
Principles, value of, 4–8, 9 fig. 1.1,
    115–18
Priorities, setting of, 21–26, 29, 73–74,
    187–88
Prodicus, 211
Punctuality, importance of, 20, 64, 93,
    173

Rabelais, François, 154–55
Reade, Charles, 219
Regius professorship at Oxford, 96, 149
Reid, Edith, 78, 93, 103, 167
Relationships, interpersonal, 174–78. *See
    also* Browne, Thomas, on interper-
    sonal relations;
  Tolerance, as personality trait
Rockefeller, John Davison, 17, 117
Role models, importance of, 3, 10, 71–72,
    134. *See also* Heroes; Mentoring
Rome, Italy, 55
Royal College of Physicians, London, 49,
    217
Royal Society of Medicine, of Great Brit-
    ain, 178
Royce, Josiah, 40

Sanderson, John Burdon, 149
Self-esteem, importance of, 158–59, 245
    n. 93, 245–46 *n.* 94
Serenity, based on acting or not acting,
    159, 160 fig. 6.1
Shakespeare, William, 29, 74, 92, 101,
    151, 165–66, 199
Socrates, 46
Speaking, as skill, 171–74
Stillé, Alfred, 21, 143
Stokes, William, 63
Stress, as cause of illness, 147–51
Student–teacher relationship. *See* Men-
    toring
Sydenham, Thomas, 69–70, 99, 111, 127,
    203

Sylvius, Franciscus, 127

Taciturnity, value of, 84, 173, 182–86.
    See also Osler, William, opinions,
    on brevity
Temperance, value of, 188–92
Tennyson, Alfred, 117
Teresa of Ávila, Saint, 209
Thayer, William Sydney, 23–24, 26, 27,
    29, 74, 114–15, 167, 173, 183
Thucydides, 12
Time management, 3–30
Time Management Matrix®, 24 fig. 1.2
Tolerance, as personality trait, 84–85
Toronto, University of, 91
Toronto Medical School, 33, 60, 63
Traits, character and personality. *See
    specific traits*; Osler, William; Osler,
    William, characteristics and traits;
    and Osler, William, opinions.
Traube, Ludwig, 119
Trinity College, Toronto, 9, 33, 60, 63
Trollope, Anthony, 184–86
Trudeau, Edward Livingston, 21, 38–39

Vaillant, George Eman, 100–101
Values, *See* Principles; Priorites
Vienna, Austria, 10, 41
Virchow, Rudolf, 10, 41, 75, 179
Voltaire [François Marie Arouet], 111

Washington, D.C., 55
Welch, William Henry, 17, 44, 89, 96,
    124, 181, 208
Weston, Ontario, 5, 60
Whitman, Walt, 156
Wilberforce, Bishop Samuel, 33
Wilson, James Cornelius, 196
Wistar, Caspar, 175–76
Women, as medical students and physi-
    cians, 36, 75, 233 *n.* 55
Woods, Hiram, 168
Work, importance of, 4, 7, 84, 90–94
World War I, 40, 103, 162–163, 215
Writing, as skill, 161–67

Yale University, 4, 47
Yeats, William Butler, 187